Table of Contents

The Authors

Mary Amdur, Ph.D., retired as Associate Professor of Toxicology, School of Public Health, Harvard University; senior Research Scientist, Energy Laboratory, Massachussets Institute of Technology and Research Professor of Environmental Medicine, Nelson Institute of Environmental Medicine, New York University.

Douglas William Dockery, B.S., M.S., Sc.D., is Associate Professor of Environmental Epidemiology, School of Public Health, and Associate Professor of Medicine (Epidemiology), Medical School, both at Harvard University.

John S. Evans, B.S.E., S.M., Sc.D., is Senior Lecturer in Environmental Science and Engineering Program, School of Public Health, Harvard University.

Petros Koutrakis, M.S., Ph.D., is Professor of Environmental Sciences in the School of Public Health, Harvard University.

A. Haluk Özkaynak, B.S., M.S., Ph.D., is Research Associate and Lecturer in Exposure Assessment and Engineering in the School of Public Health, Harvard University.

Arden Pope, Ph.D., is Professor of Economics at Brigham Young University.

Jonathan M. Samet, M.D., is Professor and Chairman of the Department of Epidemiology, School of Hygiene and Public Health, Johns Hopkins University, Baltimore, MD.

Constantine Sioutas, Sc.D., is Assistant Professor in Aerosol Engineering and Industrial Hygiene in the School of Public Health, Harvard University.

John Daniel Spengler, Ph.D., S.B., M.S, is Professor of Environmental Health in the Faculty of Public Health, Harvard University.

Mark J. Utell, M.D., is Professor of Medicine and Environmental Medicine, and Director, Pulmonary/Critical Care and Occupational Medicine Divisions, University of Rochester School of Medicine and Dentistry, Rochester, N.Y.

Richard Wilson, M.A., D.Phil., is Mallinckrodt Professor of Physics, Faculty of Arts and Sciences, and Affiliate of the Center for Risk Analysis, School of Public Health, both of Harvard University.

Scott K. Wolff, M.S., is a doctoral student at the School of Public Health, Harvard University.

The authors gratefully acknowledge the invaluable assistance of Margaret Macauley B.A, particularly in assembling Chapters 6 and 7, of Yeong Loh particularly in collecting the figures and putting them into a computer, and of Kumkum Dilwali, Ph.D., John E Yocom, P.E., C.I.H. and Sharon M. McCarthy, Ph.D., for help in drafts and collection of much of the data of Chapter 4 and Professor Terence H. Risby, Ph.D., of Johns Hopkins University for his helpful comments and suggestions during the preparation of Chapter 5.

Preface

Joseph Brain

Adults, depending on their size and physical activities, breathe tens of thousands of liters of air daily. The particles contained in this air are potentially hazardous. In this book, Drs. Spengler and Wilson and their fellow authors provide the scientific basis for a clearer understanding of this concern. A book focusing on particles in the air and their relationship to human health is both timely and important. There is considerable dispute about the causes of diseases such as diabetes, breast cancer, or cancer of the prostate. The relative role of genetics and environmental factors is not well defined. For the individual, we are unable to give clear and compelling advice with respect the successful prevention of these diseases.

In contrast, respiratory diseases such as lung cancer, emphysema, or fibrosis have been shown to be tightly linked to the environment. These diseases are caused by "particles in our air," primarily those found in cigarette smoke and in work, urban, and home environments. Most respiratory diseases are initiated and aggravated by particles and gases in the air we breathe. The lungs have a unique proximity to the environment. The same thinness and delicacy that qualify the air-blood barrier for the rapid exchange of oxygen and carbon dioxide reduce its effectiveness as a barrier to inhaled carcinogens, toxic particles, and noxious gases.

As Dr. Wilson indicates in Chapter 1, the link between particles in the air and human disease has been established many times throughout the past millennium. However, emerging global changes as well as new laboratory and epidemiological findings bring new urgency to this concern. Not only is the population growing on the planet, but there is also rapid migration to urban centers. While only 10 percent of Chinese people lived in cities in 1950, almost 50 percent of the Chinese population will live in cities by the year 2000. In addition there is growing use of cars and trucks as well as increased coal burning for industrial development and increased electric consumption in homes. There are also billions of people in Asia, Latin America, and Africa who use biomass fuels for home cooking and heating. The result is significant inhalation exposures, not only for women, but also for children, who are often closer to smoky fires because of their size.

Concern about urban particles and health is not limited to the developing world. In North America and Western Europe, many epidemiologic investigations document the relationship between ambient particulates and human health. Studies such as the Harvard Six Cities Study (Dockery, et al 1993) and many other comparable prospective and cross-sectional studies have shown that respirable particulates are associated with increased respiratory symptoms such as bronchitis, chronic cough, persistent anatomic lung disease, and fatal illness. More recently, more than a dozen studies have suggested that ambient particle concentrations can be correlated with acute mortality both in the United States and abroad. Examples include research reported by Dockery et al. (1992), Pope et al. (1992) and Schwartz (1993). Importantly, the relationship between urban particulates and mortality is a relationship that appears to be linear; there is no hint of a threshold. Moreover, this mortality effect occurs even at levels below the current United States EPA particle (PM_{10}) standard. Not surprisingly, such assertions have aroused considerable concern as well as scientific interest.

These epidemiologic findings have led to renewed interest in animal toxicology and to new experimental designs. Two testable hypotheses suggest themselves. First, the particles commonly used in contemporary human chamber or animal studies may be non-representative of "wild" urban ambient particles. Second, the healthy young animals studied may not be representative of those humans most susceptible to increased mortality in urban areas. Thus, the most appropriate animal studies may be those with concentrated ambient particles which are administered to animals with pre-existing cardiopulmonary disease.

This book clearly reflects a national and international concern about airborne particles and human health. It explores sources and characterization of airborne particles. The scope of exposure assessment extends from outdoors to a variety of indoor environments. This book also links animal studies with clinical and epidemiological studies of humans exposed to airborne particles.

Finally, this scientific information is incorporated into models and especially into public policy: what are we to make of this information as citizens? This is both timely and important. There is a growing awareness among regulatory agencies, the Congress of United States, and especially the public that particles in the air do make a difference, especially to those elderly and sick inhabitants who are most susceptible. These concerns must be quantified and expressed in environmental and occupational policy. This book is offered to the world in the hope that it will lead to the design of better experiments, to improved analysis of existing data, and to the development of creative solutions which will reduce particle exposure and the resulting health effects.

1

Introduction

Richard Wilson

Early History

As early as the ninth century, A.D., "sea-coales" were found on the northeast coast of England and burned as fuel. It was soon noticed that noxious fumes were produced upon burning, and the coal and the fumes became intolerable in the city of London. At that time there was still plenty of wood in the country so that during his reign of 1272–1307, Edward I, an early environmentalist, banned the use of "carbone marino" (sea coal) from London with the following proclamation:

> Restrictions on the use of kilns in London. The King to (the Sheriff) of Surrey, greetings. As a result of the serious complaint from the prelates and magnates of our realm, who frequently come to London for the good of the commonwealth by our order, and from the citizens and all the people who dwell there and at Southwark, we have learned that, whereas previously the makers of kilns in the aforesaid city and village and their neighborhood were in the habit of using brushwood or charcoal for their kilns, they are now again, contrary to their usual practice, firing them with and constructing them of sea-coal, from which is emitted so powerful and unbearable a stench that, as it spreads throughout the neighborhood, the air there is polluted over a wide area, to the considerable annoyance of the said prelates, magnates, citizens and others dwelling there, and to the detriment of their bodily health. Wishing to take precautions against this kind of danger, and to provide for the safety of the prelates and magnates, citizens and others of our faithful, we instruct you to have public proclamation made in the aforesaid village of

Southwark that all those who wish to operate kilns in this same village or its neighborhood should make them in the customary fashion from brushwood or charcoal and should henceforth make absolutely no use of seacoal in constructing these same kilns, under pain of heavy forfeiture. And see that this order of ours is inviolably observed hereafter throughout the aforesaid village and its neighborhood. Attested by the King at Carlisle, 12 June. In like manner an order is issued to the mayor and sheriffs of London. Attested as above. (Plantaganet 1307, as translated by Sir W. Hawthorne 1978, p. 485)

The successor to Edward I, Edward II (1307–1327) ordered persons to be tortured who were found fouling the air with coal smoke. Following the reign of Edward III, Richard II (1377–1399) adopted a more moderate position and sought to restrict the use of coal through taxation. (Many scientists are still trying to persuade governments to restrict the use by a "carbon tax." But this was rejected once more, by the U.S. Congress in summer 1993 and never even came to a vote.) Two reigns later, Henry V (1413–1422) established a commission to regulate the entry of coal into London (Chambers 1977).

By the sixteenth century, the population had increased and the woodlands cleared so that coal burning became a necessity. The court physician to Queen Elizabeth I took out a patent to remove the sulfur (Armytage 1961), but, as we all know, this process is neither cheap nor reliable even today, four centuries later. One hundred years later the problems were already very bad. The diarist John Evelyn wrote:

It is this horrid smoake, which obscures our churches and makes our palaces look old, which fouls our clothes and corrupts the waters so that the very rain and refreshing dews which fall in the several seasons precipitate this impure vapour, which with its black and tenacious quality, spots and contaminates whatever is exposed to it. (Evelyn 1661)

Burning coal produces particulate matter and sulfur oxides in the smoke, along with nitrogen oxides and their derived particles and other trace substances. For instance, it is one of the principal ways in which mercury and other heavy elements enter the atmosphere. The long-term health hazards of low levels of these metals is unknown. The amount of radioactive material—radium and thorium—is enough to make the problem of long-lived (greater than 500 years) radioactive waste from coal burning comparable to the waste from a nuclear power plant.

It is instructive to speculate on the public perception of the relative problems of sulfur and other pollution. More attention has been paid to sulfur than to nitrates; it is not entirely clear why. Sulfur certainly produces an odor; when Dante saw sulfur miners in Sicily melting the sulfur out of the ore he was inspired to write "The Inferno." Since then Hell has been composed of fire and brimstone, not fire and nitric acid. We are reminded of the prayer common in some Victorian churches in Britain: "From Hell, Hull, and Halifax, Good Lord deliver us." Whether the association of Hull and Halifax with Hell was due to air pollution is uncertain.

The Industrial Revolution was accompanied by very few pollution controls. People erected factories in places where water was available for mills. The smoke released from the chimney stacks, and from the coal-burning workers' homes nearby, often was trapped in a temperature inversion. The wealthier citizens escaped the cities either by living on the tops of hills or by using weekend houses in the country. From the beginning of the current century, however, steady improvement has been made in pollution control. The first method adopted, primarily by industry, was dispersion of the pollution by tall chimney stacks. Tall stacks had already been advocated by Evelyn (1661):

> Till more effectual methods can take place, it would be of great service, to oblige all these trades which make use of large fires, to carry their chimneys higher into the air than they are at present; this expedient would frequently help to convey the smoke way above the buildings and in a great measure disperse it into distant parts without falling on the houses below.

Early Pollution Control

Even as late as the first half of the 20th century many experts believed that tall stacks were adequate to ensure a healthy environment. For example, in a classic text, Herington (1920) says:

> It is quite true that perhaps 60 percent of the fly ash goes up through the stack. This ash is of such light fluctuant nature that it is dissipated over a wide area before precipitation occurs and no trouble can be expected from this source, although the...tonnage put out...seems great.

The next improvement was to install devices that eventually suppressed 99.5 percent by weight of the particulates, leaving mostly small aerosols to escape to the atmosphere. Unfortunately sulfur and nitrogen oxides, being gases, also escape collection by those devices designed to collect particles. But the problem was not only caused by industrial activity. Most houses in northern Europe and the United States were heated by soft coal, and the domestic burners used low chimney stacks and had no particulate, sulfur, or nitrogen oxide suppression. Transportation was by railroad run by coal-fired steam engines which blackened the neighborhood. Even as late as 1950 it was reported that in Glasgow, Scotland, three tons of soot fell per acre per year. Although the problem was not generally as bad in the United States; there are a few cities—Pittsburgh, for example—where it was as bad.

In the latter half of the 20th century, public attention was drawn to the major effects of air pollution by a number of air pollution "incidents or episodes." The first well described episode occurred when air pollutants were trapped in the Meuse Valley of Belgium during the first week of December 1930 (Firket 1931,1936) mortality and morbidity (illness) increased markedly during the days of high air pollution and for several days thereafter—many cattle and 60 people died in the first week. Firket estimated that SO_2 concentrations were in the range of 25,000–100,000 $\mu g/m^3$ (25–100 mg/m^3). Autopsy results of the victims showed only general irritation and congestion of the mucosa of the tracheas and the large bronchi in the upper respiratory tract.

The air became so hazy during the episode in Donora, Pennsylvania in October 1948, that people could not see across the street. About half the population of 14,000 became sick, 10% severely ill, and 20 deaths were attributed to the episode. (Screnck et al. 1949). Concentrations of SO_2 in the polluted air were estimated at 1,400–5,500 $\mu g/m^3$ (1.5–5.5 mg/m^3). A ten year follow-up study (Ciooco and Thompson 1961) found that those that were affected during the episode had a subsequent higher mortality rate than those not affected suggesting permanent damage of some sort.

The 1952 London Fog

In London from December 5th to 9th 1952, there was a bad fog. As was common in the autumn, a temperature inversion covered the Thames Valley and trapped air pollution for several days. Air pollution (measured somewhat inaccurately by the old British Smoke Index) suggested particulate levels as high as 4 *milligrams* per square centimeter. (Beaver 1954) When 6 months later the total death rates in London were available, a five fold increase was observed in the days starting just after the rise in air pollution, as shown in Figure 1.1 (from Beaver 1954). Already acid aerosols were suggested as a root cause. The Ministry of Health report

FIGURE 1.1

Daily Mean Pollution Concentrations and Daily Numbers of Deaths
During the London Fog Episode of 1952

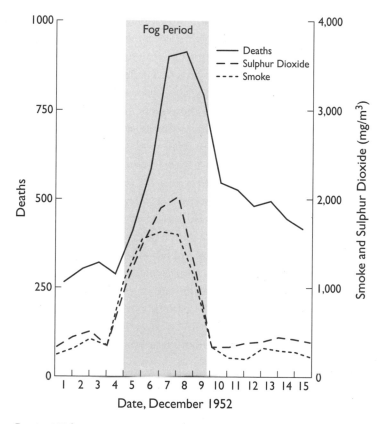

Source: Beaver, 1954

(Beaver 1954) noted that "it is probable that sulphur (sic) trioxide dissolved as sulphuric acid in fog droplets, appreciably reinforced the harmful effects of sulphur dioxide." The increase in death rate was not seen in the preceding and the following years. Few scientists now doubt that the increase in mortality in December 1952 was related to the air pollution, but most scientists believed that there is a threshold below which there is no effect. The obvious solution was to ensure that air pollution levels always remained below that threshold. The political response was immediate. The British parliament enacted the clean air act that forbad the burning of soft coal in the center of London. The implementation of this, and other clean air acts was aided by the availability of cheap oil and natural gas from the Persian/Arabian Gulf and the North Sea. As a result of this act and its implementation, many of the particulate emitters in London are no longer close to ground level, but are the tall chimney stacks that send the pollution above the inversion layer, and far out to sea. The current concern is from mobile source emission—often burning diesel fuels for which the tall stack solution is impossible.

The government-mandated cleanup has been impressive and obvious. Although a bad fog occurred again in 1962, the death rate increase was smaller than in 1952—less than twice the normal death rate (Commins and Waller 1967). In this incident there were better measurements and acid aerosols were also elevated—an indication of a possible root cause that will be discussed in several chapters of the book. But by 1980 the bad fogs in London and Pittsburgh that persisted until 1950 had disappeared. By sending pollution above the inversion layer, even the local weather changed. Until recently, most experts considered that these measures were all the pollution control that is necessary. But by 1980 new health and property damage assessments, and a general rise of standards and expectations, suggested that maybe society should do more to ensure clean air. The local problem had been solved but it soon appeared that a global one may have replaced it. Particulate levels rose in the countryside as the pollution was spread. More insidious, perhaps, is that the particulate control in the tall chimneys removed the larger particles but allowed many of the finer ones to remain. These fine particles stayed airborne for longer than the heavy particles, and when finally reaching ground level were in the range that could be readily inhaled.

Lave and Seskin Studies

In a seminal set of papers written by Lave and Seskin (1970, 1971, 1972, 1973, 1977) an "association" between air pollution variables and death rates in a number of United States air quality districts was described. The association was largest with particulates not with sulfur dioxide. This association was immediately doubted. If air pollution levels had visibly, and measurably, been vastly improved, how could there be such an effect? Even the details of the computation were questioned. Over a period of ten years the *arithmetic* was confirmed and the analysis was refined and extended to include more recent morbidity and data on pollutant concentrations by a number of other investigators, (Evans, Tosteson and Kinney 1984, Özkaynak and Thurston 1987) but causality was still unclear. Associations were also found between daily morbidity and mortality and daily air pollution variables. These were smaller than the obvious associations of Figure 1.1, but still appeared to be statistically significant. But other explanations seemed likely. Leonard, Crowley and Benton (1950) had analyzed deaths from respiratory disease in Dublin from 1938 to 1949. These showed a diurnal variation of death rate which appeared to correlate with increases in particulate air pollution. But death rate variations continued even when after 1941 air pollution was reduced and correlated with season. Air pollution was associated with winter weather and winter weather keeps people indoors where both the spread of infectious diseases and air pollution may be different from that out of doors.

Moreover even in the London air pollution incidents a puzzle arose. It was publicly stated and widely believed, that the effect of air pollution was primarily that sick people died somewhat earlier than otherwise. If that were true, one would expect an effect known as "harvesting." The increase in mortality in the second week of December 1952 should have been accompanied by a decrease in the following month or so (the decrease should show up in the plot of Figure 1.1 as a dip of the same area as the increase in the earlier week). On the contrary the death rate remained somewhat high for some weeks after the episode and this behavior was repeated in 1962. If the overall effect had been small, so that causality would not be so obvious, it would be considered to be a reason for believing that the effect itself is spurious. Some authors find significant negative "auto-correlations," (Spix et al. 1994, Wyzga and Lipfert 1995b, Cifuentes and Lave 1996) which are consistent with the harvesting hypothesis. This is often brought up by those who doubt that air pollution still has an adverse effect but this puzzle has never been quantitatively explained (Wyzga 1977).

In Lave and Seskin's studies there seemed to be no clear cut (specific) medical end result, and moreover Lave and Seskin had performed *linear* regressions, thereby implying a linear dose response relationship. This encouraged the doubters, many of whom believed that any real effect would not exist at some safe level, and increase rapidly above a threshold. On the other hand there were other scientists who felt that a linear dose response is not only possible, but likely. It would be nice if we could distinguish definitively between the two limits of a firm threshold model, and a proportional incidence model by direct observation or experiment. This is not possible, largely because the effects of air pollution on death rate are delayed, and causality is hard to establish.

It is not possible to rigorously prove the existence or absence of a threshold even for tobacco cigarette smoking, which kills five to ten times as many Americans (approximately 300,000 per year) as the worst estimates of air pollution. We know from the work of Doll and Peto (1976) that smoking four cigarettes a day gives about one-tenth the incidence of lung cancer among British physicians as smoking 40 cigarettes a day, yet we cannot directly tell whether or not one cigarette a week is harmful, although it does appear probable that living with a smoker and inhaling second hand "side-stream" smoke increases the cancer risk slightly. We can compare directly a smoker with his neighbor who is exposed to similar amounts of other pollutants, so that an epidemiologic assessment is possible. We cannot easily find large matched groups of those exposed to air pollutants and those not so exposed. Much more serious is that as we mitigate the known and obvious effects of air pollution, we are led to disperse the pollutant sources and dilute the pollutants, making the task of comparison harder.

The work of Lave and Seskin and others also had another serious problem. They studied a possible statistical association between death rates averaged over an air pollution quality district and a measure of outdoor air pollution averaged over this district. This is called an "Ecological study." All too often scientists try to obtain more information than is possible from such a study. The major error is often called the "Ecological Fallacy." We would prefer to have an association between an individual probability of death and individual measures of air pollution, with individual estimates of the major confounding influences such as cigarette smoking. As a result many, if not most epidemiologists regarded the suggestion that air pollution caused respiratory deaths as unproven at best, and untrue at worst. The implications of the ecological fallacy in a similar problem—disentangling the risk of lung cancer caused by low concentrations of radon gas in the presence of a much larger risk of lung cancer caused by cigarette smoking has been addressed by Stidley and Samet (1993, 1994). Their cautionary words are applicable here.

Such was the situation in 1980 when the first edition of this book was printed (Wilson et al. 1980). We had little hope that we would ever have much more reliable data. We therefore collected together data on animal tests, tests of metabolism, and theoretical ideas. In Figure 1.2 we show a chart showing the health effects of SO_2 and particulates as they were then understood. In the bottom left hand corner was a region labelled "NO EFFECT." We alter this to read "EFFECT ONLY SEEN IN LARGE POPULATIONS." In the intervening 17 years, there have been extensive animal tests on combustion products, and there is more supporting evidence that fine (<2.5 µm), acid, particulates can be detrimental to the respiratory tract and may be causing large (3% increase of the age adjusted

FIGURE 1.2

Dose Response Curve for Sulfur Dioxide and Total Suspended Particulates

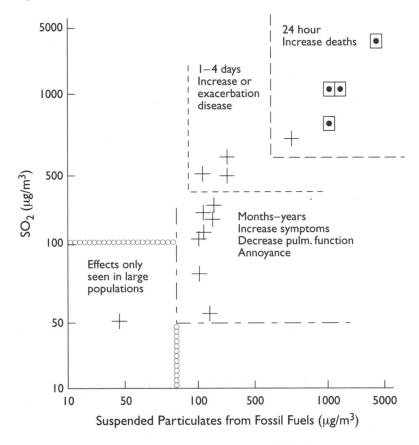

death rate) effects on health. In addition there have now been two cohort studies relating the respiratory deaths of specific people in cohorts of people exposed. These cohort studies are less liable to error than the previous ecological studies.

The New Evidence

Recent reports of an association between levels of particles in outdoor air and daily mortality counts have again raised concern that air pollution causes deaths that would not have occurred if pollution were not present. Concern that outdoor air pollution increases mortality had largely abated by the late 1970s, following the introduction of air pollution control measures and the decline of pollution levels in the United States, the United Kingdom, and other countries (Holland et al. 1979). The initial evidence that air pollution could increase mortality came from well-chronicled and dramatic pollution episodes, like the London Fog of 1952, during which obvious increases in death counts were observed.

It is the purpose of this book to describe the new evidence within the last 15 years in the words of the investigators themselves, yet in a coherent way. Much that was in the first edition that is irrelevant to this theme (effect of CO_2 on global warming; effects of radionuclides, sulfur dioxide control) is omitted.

In Chapter 2 we discuss the *nature* of the aerosols and particles in the ambient air, with some concentration on the fine particles that are believed to cause some adverse health effects. In this chapter also is a discussion of the measurement methods available to assess the *concentrations* of air pollutants. All too often emphasis is placed upon the *emissions* of the pollutants, whereas which are less closely related to any effects upon health.

Chapter 3 discusses the emissions, the dispersion and the concentrations of particles. We enumerate the emissions of particles in the U.S. and describe how the anthropogenic (caused by human activity) airborne particulates are related to the natural ones. We will describe the nature of the particles that are emitted from various sources and the way they transmute in the atmosphere; sulfur dioxide gas, for example, can attach to particles or moisture droplets to become acid particulates. Fine particles, emitted at the top of tall chimney stack, can be carried by the wind for thousands of miles. However, because an adequate monitoring system does not exist to fully characterize air pollutant concentrations, we also briefly describe how air dispersion calculations may be used to calculate concentrations from known emission sources.

Chapter 4 discusses the personal exposure to particles, which exposure is responsible for the *dose* of particles that enter, and stay in the lung. We do not measure this dose, but infer the dose from the *exposure* to the air pollutants, combined with an estimate of the air volume breathed. The exposure, could in principle be measured with a personal monitor, but more often is inferred from a measure of *outdoor concentration plus an assumption about* occupancy. Although the initial comparisons of the concentrations of air pollutants indoors and outdoors suggested large differences, it will be shown in Chapter 4 that there is little difference between indoor and outdoor concentrations of the smaller size particulates that are now suggested to be of major concern. (d<1 μm) This point is crucial; unless the measure of outdoor air pollution is a good surrogate for the actual exposure it is reasonable to question the causal nature of the associations found.

Chapter 5 will describe how laboratory animals, particularly guinea pigs, display bronchial constriction when they inhale pollutants and that the constriction is greater when the inhaled particles are acid and are small (<3.5 μm). These studies, begun intensively after the air pollution incidents were recorded, told us very early that a problem was likely. There is a strong indication of a linear relation between response (constriction of airways) and dose. This response is not, in itself usually considered a major adverse health response but the connection is made in later chapters. Reduction in pulmonary function can increase the probability of other, worse, effects on health.

Chapter 6 will describe the many recent, careful, epidemiological studies relating acute effects, both deaths and morbidity, from respiratory diseases to air pollution variables, as a function of time (time series studies). These are the "acute" effects that occur soon after exposure. The early time series studies found a larger death rate in winter, when the air pollution is high, than in the summer, when air pollution is less, which is no longer true in the U.S. so that the role of winter factors as a confounder has changed. The techniques of smoothing temperature extremes by Schimmel have been extended and improved. Other winter factors, staying indoors and spreading disease, or cold, can obviously confuse the results. It is largely in separating such confounding variables that the recent epidemiological studies are improvements upon the early ones. The increase in the number of locations and situations studied vastly reduces the likelihood of confounders.

While many of the early epidemiological studies related death rates with sulfur pollution, especially sulfur dioxide (SO_2 pollution) more recent ones in the U.S. have found stronger correlations with particulates, and especially the "fine" fraction. Usually the PM_{10} (<10 μm) fraction was discussed although the $PM_{3.5}$ (<3.5 μm) fraction, or even the $PM_{2.5}$ (<2.5 μm) fraction, is now believed to be more important. Figure 1.3 (from Lippmann 1985) shows how the coefficient relating annual mortality to ambient air pollution (relative to the sulfate component) becomes larger and more statistically significant as one proceeds from Total Suspended Particles (TSP) to Inhalable Particles (IP) and then to fine Particles (FP). This might be expected to improve further if the truly causative air pollution variable were found. However, the acidity of the particulates, and in particular the relationship to sulfuric acid, has unfortunately NOT been a directly measured air pollution variable and has to be inferred indirectly.

FIGURE 1.3

Schematic (Due to Lippman) Showing How an Estimated Effect on Mortality Increases (and Might Increase Further) When Plotted Against a Surrogate that Approaches the True Root Cause

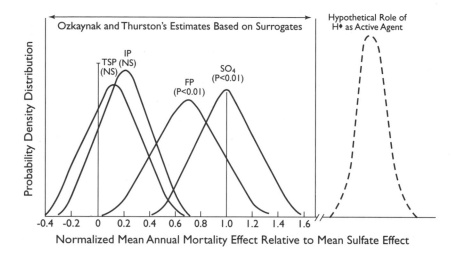

The associations have been found using new statistical methods for time series data: primarily Poisson regression models which are fit to the data using methods like the generalized estimating equations of Liang and Zeger (Liang and Zeger 1986) which can account for inherent difficulties posed by time series data. Modeling approaches have been questioned (Moolgavkar et al. 1995), although the findings have proved robust and not sensitive to choice of analytical methods (EPA 1995, Schwartz 1994, Camilli et al. 1987). However when several air pollution variables vary together (are colinear) epidemiological studies *by themselves* cannot distinguish which is the true causative agent (Moolgavkar and Luebeck 1996). Animal data of Chapter 5 or human experimental studies of Chapter 8 must be used. These suggest, for example, that particles are more likely to be causative agents than SO_2 gas.

Chapter 7 will describe how the same air pollution can lead to effects which are long delayed (chronic effects). These associations are revealed by relating health effects as a function of ambient air pollution experienced at different locations (cross-sectional studies). The cross sectional studies show higher death rates in cities than in the countryside. The increase in diseases associated with the respiratory system, such as lung cancer, show the largest associations. The epidemiologist in these studies must address the many confounding factors associated with urban life. The coefficient relating the health effect to a pollution variable should, and does, become greater, and less uncertain, the closer the variable is to that directly causing the pollution. This is illustrated in Figure 1.3.

Chapter 8 describes the experiments on controlled human exposure to pollutant gases and aerosols. These human experiments have been guided both by the animal studies described in Chapter 5, and by the epidemiological studies. These human experiments can only, by their nature, be of short term duration and therefore address the *acute* epidemiological findings of Chapter 6 more than the *chronic* epidemiological findings of Chapter 7. The epidemiology findings at low exposures appears discordant with our understanding of how inhaled particles could adversely affect health (Utell and Samet 1993, Utell and Frampton 1995).

In this chapter is a discussion of possible mechanisms by which air pollutants might affect people. This chapter is important because two research physicians discuss the biological, toxicological and medical conditions required of any biologically plausible model.

Chapter 9 is a partial response to the challenge of proving biological plausibility. It describes a first attempt to create a plausible mathematical *model* for studies presented in Chapter 7. A mathematical (statistical) model is presented that could account for the observed associations. Noting that the observed associations are with diseases related to the respiratory system, we suggest a model that the fine particulates cause damage to the lung, often irreversible, that reduces lung function roughly in proportion to the dose. For the healthy young the effect on lung function is small and does not appreciably affect the ability to function, or health generally. For a person with ailments, or merely in old age, this reduction may be enough to be the "last straw" in causing effects upon health. To the extent that such a model is correct, it is possible to derive consequences which can be tested in other situations.

Chapter 10 discusses various public policy issues and questions that are raised by the data. If it were cheap and easy to avoid the air pollution it would have been done, and the scientists and others who believe that there is a threshold would not have objected. But that is not the case. There is no cheap way to avoid the pollution. There must be a trade off. If the number of victims of air pollution is zero, and all of the money spent upon remediation would be wasted. Moreover, the rising costs of electricity from pollutant control could give secondary adverse health effects. This is calculated from a general maxim "wealthier is healthier." This was been stressed only a few years ago by McCarroll (1979), who obviously did not believe the idea that ambient concentrations caused adverse heath effects, in the following paragraph.

All these health costs (due to increased electricity costs) are real and must be balanced against any anticipated benefit from reduced SO_x levels achieved by costly scrubbing of stack effluents, or by burning of expensive desulfurized fuel. Since no detectable excess mortality can be found ascribable to SO_2 or sulfates at presently prevailing levels, money used to reduce these levels still further might better be used for other public health purposes.

Even though animal data, auxiliary to the epidemiology data suggest that it is the very fine particles, probably with acid and/or metals adsorbed on the surfaces, that are responsible for the association, there still remains great difficulty in being sure exactly what is, or are, the causative agents (Lipfert and Wyzga 1995). It is therefore not easy to be sure what appropriate remedial actions to take. A general action such as reducing all fossil fuel burning will, however, be effective independent of the specific cause.

These conclusions are described as a National Dilemma for the U.S., and also discuss some international ramifications. To what extent are the conclusions applicable to developing countries where particle pollution is often worse than what was experienced in Europe and the U.S. over the first six decades of this century?

The focus of the first edition was on sulfur oxides (SO_x), nitrogen oxides (NO_x), and particulates; or colloquially, SOCKS, KNOCKS and ROCKS. In this edition the focus is narrowed; it is upon fine, respirable, acid particulates, and more particularly sulfuric acid particulates, perhaps sorbed on trace metal particulates such as zinc or iron oxides.

2

Physico-Chemical Properties and Measurement of Ambient Particles

Petros Koutrakis and Constantinos Sioutas

Introduction

Atmospheric aerosols are complex mixtures of particles directly emitted into the atmosphere and particles that are formed during gas-to-particle conversion processes. The sources of atmospheric particles are both natural and anthropogenic. Particle size is the most important parameter in describing particle behavior and the origin, chemical and composition, removal, and residence time in the atmosphere are all related to the particle size. This chapter discusses the origin and the main characteristics of atmospheric aerosols. Particle formation and removal processes are presented. The main particle characterization methods, including direct-reading and integrated sampling instruments, are discussed. A presentation of the most common analytical methods to determine particle chemical composition is also included.

Ambient aerosols are defined as suspensions of relatively stable solid or liquid particles in the surrounding air. Generally, the term refers to the particulate matter, although the "strict" definition includes both suspended matter and the surrounding air. There are several ways to classify aerosols. The major distinction is that between primary and seondary aerosols. Primary aerosols consist of particles directly emitted into the atmosphere, whereas secondary aerosols consist of particles that are products of gas-to-particle conversion processes. Aerosols are also classified according to their sources into natural and anthropogenic aerosols. Table 2.1 shows the principal sources of natural and anthropogenic aerosols. The physical and chemical characteristics of aerosols are strongly dependent on the type of their formation mechanisms and sources as shown in Figure 2.1. On a small scale, the dynamics of primary aerosols are

FIGURE 2.1

Schematic of an atmospheric aerosol size distribution showing the three modes, the main source of mass in each mode, and the principal processes involved in inserting mass into and removing mass from each mode.

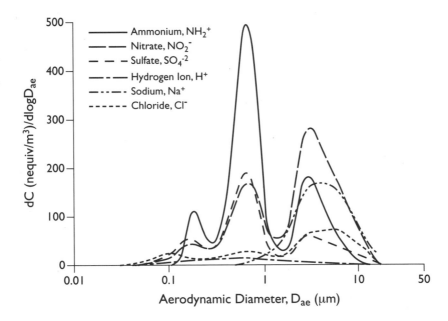

From Wang and John, 1988. Reproduced with permission, Copyright © Elsevier Science Inc., 1988.

influenced by Brownian diffusion and coagulation, and on a large scale by atmospheric mixing processes. Aerosol properties are subjected to continuous changes through a number of chemical and physical processes. For example, natural sodium chloride (NaCl) particles react with anthropogenic sulfuric acid (H_2SO_4) to form Na_2SO_4 particles.

The different mechanisms of formation also influence the size distribution of ambient aerosols (Whitby 1980). Ambient particles range from 0.01 to 100 μm in diameter. The particle size range from 0.01 to 0.1 μm is known as the "ultrafine mode," or "Aitken nuclei mode." These particles have relatively short residence times in the atmosphere because they are physically mobile due to their Brownian diffusive motion. They are products of homogeneous nucleation of supersaturated vapors (SO_2, NH_3, NO_x, and combustion products).

T A B L E   2 . 1
Sources of Aerosols

Natural

1	Sea spray residue
2	Windblown mineral dust
3	Volcanic effluvia (includes both direct particle emissions and particles produced by subsequent reactions of emitted gases)
4	Biogenic materials (particles emitted directly and particles produced from condensation of volatile organic compounds emitted by plants)
5	Smoke from the burning of land biota
6	Natural gas-to-particle conversion products (e.g., sulfate generated from reduced sulfur emitted from the ocean surface, marshes, etc)

Anthropogenic

1	Direct anthropogenic particle emissions (e.g., soot, smoke, road dust, etc.)
2	Products of the conversion of anthropogenic gases from combustion of fossil fuels (e.g., sulfate and nitrate formed from oxidation of SO_2 and NO_2, respectively)

Source: Prospero et al. 1981

The size range 0.1 to 2.5 μm is known as the "accumulation mode" or "fine mode." They are formed by coagulation of ultrafine mode particles and through gas-to-particle conversion processes known as heterogeneous nucleation, and by condensation of gases onto pre-existing particles in the accumulation mode. The major constituents of these particles in the industrialized countries are sulfate (SO_4^{2-}), nitrate (NO_3^-), ammonium (NH_4^+), elemental (EC) and organic (OC) carbon. In addition they contain a variety of trace metals formed in combustion processes. Sulfate, nitrate, and ammonium are products of gas-to-particle conversion of sulfur dioxide (SO_2), nitrogen oxides (NO_x), and ammonia (NH_3). A host of viable species can also be present, such as fungi, bacteria, pollen, yeasts, and viruses. Fine particles are, in general, too small to settle out (by gravity) and too large to coagulate into larger particles, and thus they have lifetimes in the atmosphere of the order of days and can be transported over long distances.

The most important factor in removal of large particles from the lower atmosphere, or troposphere, is gravitational settling. In the particle range of approximately 1–20 μm the "speed of sedimentation," or terminal settling, is given by Stokes' law. Stokes described the competition between two forces acting on the particles, the resistance of the air to the particle's motion through it, which is proportional to diameter, and the force of gravity, which is proportional to the particle mass (or the cube of the diameter). The formula for the settling velocity v becomes:

$$v = \frac{d^2 \rho g}{18\eta} \tag{2-1}$$

where (in cgs units):

  v = the terminal settling velocity (cm/sec)
  ρ = particle density (g/cm^3)
  g = acceleration caused by gravity (981 cm/s^2)
  d = particle diameter (cm); and
  η = kinematic viscosity of air (1.8 x 10^{-4} poise)

It should be noted that the atmospheric residence time, which is roughly proportional to the inverse of the terminal settling velocity, varies as the inverse square of particle diameter. Stokes' law also governs the removal of particles by the electrostatic or centrifugal dust suppressors in use today. These suppressors act by increasing the acceleration of the particles above that caused by gravity. The constant g in Stokes' equation is replaced by a larger value so that the settling velocity onto the collecting surface is greater than gravity provides. However, the settling velocity still varies as the square of the particle diameter, thus although the removal efficiency for the total mass may be impressively high (i.e., 99.5 percent), the removal efficiency for the all-important respirable particles is much lower.

Particles in the size range 2.5 to 100 μm are referred to as coarse particles. These particles primarily contain soil and sea salt elements, such as Si, Al, Ca, Fe, Mn, Sr, Na, and K. They are produced by mechanical processes (grinding, erosion, or resuspension by the wind). They are relatively large, settle out of the atmosphere by gravity within hours or minutes and are only found near the source depending on height of release.

Figure 2.2 (Jaenicke 1980) shows the residence time of aerosols as a function of size and location in the atmosphere. Note that the residence time increases with the altitude, and also depends on a number of factors, such as the vertical distribution of water vapor which affects reactivity and removal processes and the vertical distribution of reactive chemical species. Particle size is the most important property of aerosols because it influences the lifetime of particles in the atmosphere, thus their effects on the environment and public health. These effects will be presented in more detail in the next section.

FIGURE 2.2

The Residence Time of Individual Particles as a Function of Particle Size and Altitude

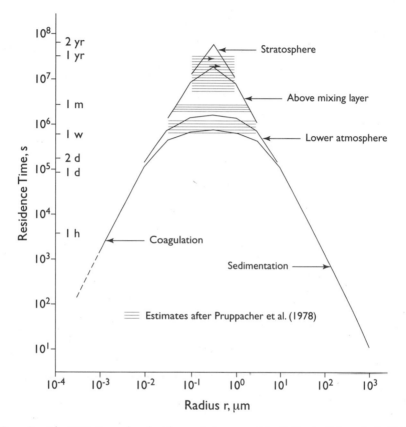

From Jaenicke 1980. Reproduced with permission, copyright © Elsevier Science Ltd., 1980

The Importance of Studying Atmospheric Aerosols
Environmental Impact

Atmospheric aerosols are important in the spatial distribution of sub-stances of environmental importance. Mineral dust from arid areas is trans-ported through aerosols to the oceans (Junge 1979, Burcher 1983). Trace elements, such as Pb, Hg, Cu, Sn, Cd, etc, are also transported by ambi-ent aerosols, resulting in significant concentrations of such compounds in long distances from their sources (Rhan 1981). Removal of these materials through dry or wet deposition mechanisms results in high concentrations in soils (Romero 1982). The chemical composition of the ocean micro-layer is also affected by atmospheric aerosols (Buat-Menard 1982).

Particle Characterization

Sampling of atmospheric particles is a complicated task and over the past twenty years one of the main goals of environmental scientists has been to improve instrumentation for determining the properties and concentrations of ambient particles. There are two main strategies for sampling and analysis of atmospheric particles, namely direct and integrated sampling.

Direct-Reading Instruments

Direct-reading instruments provide instantaneous information on the concentration and size distribution of aerosols. In these instruments, the aerosol is drawn into a "sensing" region (Swift 1989). The presence of particles gives rise to a change in some property of the sensing region, which is a function of a property of the sampled aerosol. It must be noted that these instruments provide information on particle size, as well as number and mass concentration. Traditionally, these instruments have been placed into four broad categories (First 1989): optical, electrical, resonance oscillation, and beta attenuation.

Optical counters make use of the interaction between light and particles. The theory of optical aerosol behavior and its application to particle measurement is discussed by Hodkinson (1966) and Willeke and Liu (1976). Most of the optical systems count light pulses scattered from particles that flow, one by one, through an intensely illuminated zone. Sampling flow rate is low, and the smallest detectable particle size is about 0.3 µm. The use of laser beams has made it possible to count particles as small as approximately 0.1 µm (Knollenberg and Luehr 1976), although the manufacturers recommend that concentrations higher than 100 particles per cm^3 should not be exceeded.

Electrical counters are based on charging the sampled aerosols and measuring the ability of particles to traverse an electrical field. Most of these counters draw particles through a cloud of either unipolarly or bipolarly charged ions, and each of the particles acquire a quantity of charge that is simply related to its size. Subsequently, the particles are drawn into a radially symmetric electrical field where particles smaller than a certain size, which depends on the intensity of the field, are collected onto the walls of the collecting device. By changing the field voltage, the particle size distribution can be obtained (Liu and Pui 1975, Whitby 1976).

When particles are deposited on an oscillating surface, the resonant frequency is a function of the mass collected on the surface. This is the principle on which resonant oscillation aerosol mass monitors are based. Most of the particle collection surfaces have piezoelectric properties. The oscillation frequency decreases as the mass loading increases, with the change proportional to the airborne mass concentration and the rate at which air is sampled through the instrument (Lundgren et al. 1976). Another instrument in this category is the tapered element oscillating microbalance (TEOM; Pataschnink and Rupprecht 1991). Aerosol is deposited on a filter which is placed on top of a tapered glass element which oscillates naturally. The deposition of particulate mass causes a decrease in the frequency, measured continuously by the oscillation amplifier.

Mass concentration of airborne particles can also be detected by attenuating beta radiation. In such instruments, aerosols are drawn through an orifice and impact on a surface positioned between a beta source and a counter (Macias and Husar 1976). One of the main drawbacks of this method is that attenuation may not be only a function of the collected mass (for instance, the chemical composition of the collected material may be an important factor).

In addition to the limitations specified above for these direct reading instrument methods, there are performance limitations due to some or all of the following factors: humidity, gas adsorption, and particle collection efficiency.

Integrated Samplers

Filters. Collection on a filter is the simplest method for determining particle concentration and chemical composition. A number of factors, such as filter density, porosity, pH, and composition, play an important role in its performance characteristics. The choice of filters depends on the chemical species to be analyzed, as well as the type of the analytical method to be used. For example, when measuring particle mass, the filter material must be non-hygroscopic, so that the net mass change before and after sampling is not affected by the ambient humidity. Another case is for trace metal analysis by XRF or neutron activation, the filter itself must be virtually free from the metals being measured. In general, aerosol sampling filters should meet the following criteria (Lippmann 1989): the collection efficiency should be above 90% for all particle sizes; they should be able to withstand sampling, transport and analysis processes; they should present low resistance to different extraction processes so that the collected particulate matter is easily removed; they should also present low blank concentrations. Table 2.2 (Stevens 1984) shows different types of filters widely used for ambient aerosol sampling.

The simplicity of the filter techniques is a major advantage for particle sampling, but there are still potential artifacts associated with these methods. These artifacts can result in an underestimation (negative artifact) or overestimation (positive artifact) of the concentration of particles and are due to phenomena such as the following:

▪ Acid gas phase compounds, such as SO_2, HNO_3, and a variety of organic compounds, can be adsorbed on filter media. The high retention of atmospheric sulfur and nitrogen oxides on filter media led to measurements of atmospheric nitrate and sulfate that were too high (Coutant 1977, Appel 1984). In laboratory studies, glass fiber filters were found to retain 8–21% of the SO_2 as sulfate on the filter at 21°C and 80% relative humidity, whereas quartz and Teflon retained 5% or less. This retention is related to the filter alkalinity with the most alkaline filters retaining the greatest amount of SO_2.

Adsorption of gas phase HNO_3 onto the filter medium gives a considerable artifact nitrate on certain types of filters, leading to an overestimation of particulate-phase nitrates. In laboratory studies, glass fiber filters retained more than 94% of the gaseous HNO_3 of the sampled air, while quartz filters tested retained from 33 to 99%. Only

TABLE 2.2

Properties of Filter Media Used in Ambient Aerosol Sampling

Filter and Chemical Composition	Density (mg/cm^2)	pH	Efficiency %[*]
Teflon Membrane (several manufacturers) $(CF_2)_n$ (2 µm pore size)	0.5	Neutral	99.95
Cellulose (Whatman 41) $(C_6H_{10}O_5)_n$	8.7	Neutral (reacts with HNO_3)	58.0 at 0.3 µm
Glass Fiber (Whatman GF/C)	5.16	Basic (pH=9)	99.0
Quartz (Gelman)	6.51	Neutral	98.5
Polycarbonate (Nuclepore) $C_{15}H_{14}$	0.8	Neutral	93.9
Cellulose Acetate/Nitrate (Millipore)	5.0	Neutral (reacts with HNO_3)	99.6

[*] Minimum efficiency for particle diameter > 0.035 at face velocity of 10 cm/s
Source: Stevens 1984

Teflon filters adsorbed negligible amounts of gaseous HNO_3 (Shaw et al. 1982). Even when the HNO_3 is not adsorbed to the filter material, it can react with previously collected alkaline material, particularly if the coarse alkaline particles are not separated from the fine particles.

■ Adsorption of vapor-phase organic compounds on quartz filters, resulting in an overestimation of the particulate phase, has been demonstrated in several laboratory studies (McDow et al. 1990, Fitz 1987).

■ Particle interactions on the filter media during and after sampling, such as reactions of fine particle (< 2.5 µm) acidic sulfates with coarse (> 2.5 µm) alkaline particles such as $CaCO_3$, and salts such as NaCl, or NH_4NO_3,, can form neutral sulfate salts and acid gases such as CO_2, HCl, or HNO_3. Such interactions between coarse and fine particles can be minimized by removal of the coarse particles using inertial impactors (see below). On the other hand, interactions between different types of fine particles collected on the same filter can be a more challenging problem.

■ Volatilization of unstable ammonium particulate salts, such as NH_4NO_3, and NH_4Cl, forms NH_3 and HNO_3, or HCl (Koutrakis et al. 1992). The produced ammonia can diffuse to the collected acid sulfate particles and neutralize them, as described in the previous paragraph. The produced acidic gases can be collected by coated filters of the filter pack that are placed downstream of the particle collection filter. Thus, the gas phase concentrations would depend on the amounts that existed in the atmosphere during sampling plus the amounts that volatilized from the collected particles, resulting in an overestimation of the concentration of acidic gases and an underestimation of acidic particles. Volatilization of material from collected particles during sampling has also been observed for a number of semi-volatile organic compounds. Schwartz et al. (1981) showed that moderately polar compounds were increasingly difficult to recover as the sampling period became progressively longer. Similar observations were made by Appel et al. (1984) for semi-volatile organic compounds.

Conventional and Virtual Inertial Impactors. Conventional inertial impactors have been used in several studies to determine the size distribution of ambient particles (Ahlberg et al. 1978, Wang and John 1988, Pierson et al. 1989, Koutrakis et al. 1993). In these devices particles are separated from the air sample due to their inertia. In a conventional flat plate impactor (Figure 2.3), particle-laden air passes through a nozzle where particles are accelerated. At the nozzle exit, the air streamlines are deflected sharply, so that particles larger than a certain aerodynamic size (the impactor's cut-off size) impinge on the collection surface, whereas smaller particles escape and follow the deflected streamlines. By employing more than one stage, the aerosol sample can be fractionated in several size intervals. This system is called a cascade impactor (Figure 2.4). The collected particles can be subsequently analyzed to determine their chemical composition. The nature of the impaction substrate depends on the species and the type of chemical analysis to be performed. For instance, when sampling particulate sulfate, the collection medium used as impaction surface is typically a Teflon filter, chosen for its low background acid and sulfate concentrations. For analysis of organic particles, the collection substrate is typically aluminum foil (McMurry and Zhang 1989).

Due to the extensive theoretical work (Marple and Liu 1974, Marple and Willeke 1976) the performance of conventional inertial impactors is

FIGURE   2 . 3

Schematic Diagram of a Conventional Impactor

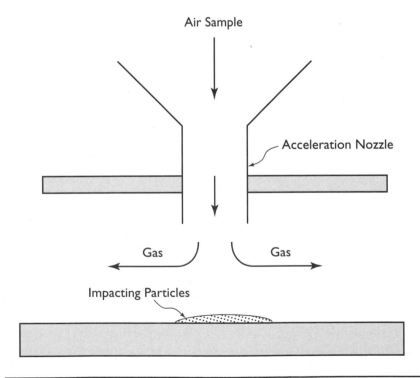

FIGURE 2.4
Schematic Diagram of a Cascade Impactor

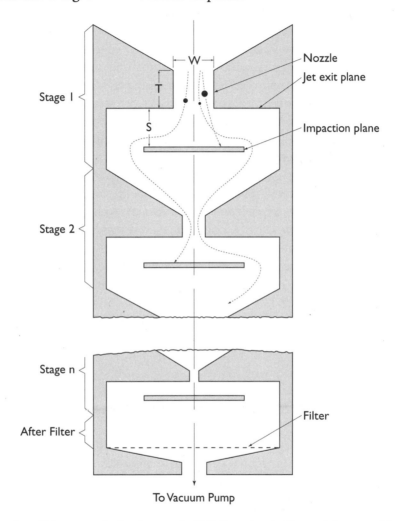

From *Aerosol Measurement* by Lundgren et al., 1976. Reproduced with permission, copyright © University Press of Florida, 1976.

well understood and their characteristics can be predicted quite accurately. These impactors can typically classify particles larger than a few tenths of a micrometer in diameter, operating at atmospheric pressure and having jets fabricated by conventional machining.

To classify smaller aerosol particles, low-pressure and microorifice impactors. Low-pressure impactors resemble ordinary impactors but operate at reduced pressures (0.05 to 0.4 atmospheres). These devices take advantage of the decreased aerodynamic drag on particles that occurs when the mean free path in the air is as large or larger than that of the particle diameter (Hering et al. 1978). These impactors operate at sampling flow rates up to 30 liters/minute.

Microorifice impactors reduce the impactor's cut-off size by accelerating particles through small diameter jet orifices (Marple et al. 1991). Microorifice impactors operate at pressures closer to atmospheric (0.7 to 0.9 atmospheres), and achieve cut points on the order of 0.1 μm by employing orifices 0.004 to 0.02 cm in diameter. Operation with a low pressure drop is very important, since evaporation of volatile compounds from the separated particles can result in a severe distortion of the size distribution (Biswas et al. 1987). Water loss could cause a decrease in the particle size. On the other hand, aerodynamic cooling within the high speed jet can cause particle size to increase by condensation of water vapor.

The most important limitations of these conventional inertial impactors are the following (Biswas et al. 1987): i) particles may bounce from the collection surface upon impaction; ii) collected particles may re-entrain; iii) wall losses between the impactor stages may be considerable; and iv) very large particles may break up upon impaction, especially at high impaction velocities. The particle bounce problem has been traditionally countered by coating the impaction plates with a sticky material. However, for certain analytical techniques, carbon-containing coatings which are typically used may interfere with the measurement of organic compounds.

Virtual inertial impactors provide an alternative solution to the particle bounce and re-entrainment problems associated with conventional impactors. Virtual impactors also classify particles according to their aerodynamic size (Figure 2.5). In this device, an acceleration nozzle (jet) directs particle-laden air toward a collection probe, which is slightly larger than the jet. Particles larger than a certain size (defined as the impactor's cut point) cross the air streamlines, due to their inertia, and enter the collection probe, whereas smaller particles follow the deflected streamlines. In order for the larger particles to enter the collection probe, a fraction of the total flow is allowed to pass through the probe, referred to as the minor flow (typically 10–20% of the total flow). As a result, the concentration of the larger particles in the minor flow has increased by a factor of Q_{tot}/Q_{min}, where Q_{tot} is the total flow entering the virtual impactor and Q_{min} is the minor flow. Most virtual impactors have the intrinsic disadvantage that the minor flow contains a small fraction (Q_{min}/Q_{tot}) of

FIGURE   2.5
Schematic Diagram of a Virtual Impactor

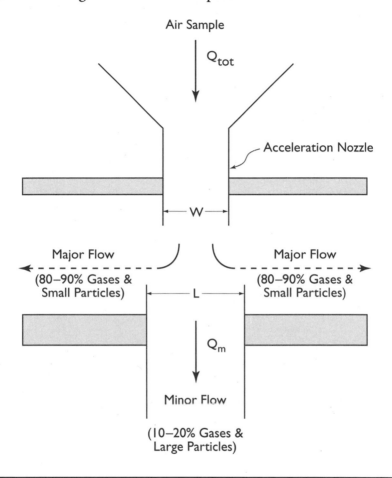

the fine particles, as a result of pumping the coarse particle flow through the collection probe. In addition, for the same flow rate, virtual impactors have less sharp size cut-off curves than conventional impactors. Masuda et al. (1988) has developed a virtual impactor with reduced fine particle contamination of the minor flow by confining the aerosol flow within a core using an enveloping sheath of clean air. Theoretical studies of the virtual impactors are similar to those of conventional impactors (Marple and Chien 1980). The dichotomous sampler (Loo et al. 1976) has been probably the most widely used virtual impactor. It has a cut point equal to 2.5 m and fractionates coarse from fine ambient particles.

In addition to the elimination of the particle bounce and re-entrainment problem, the virtual impactors have the advantage of keeping the collected particles airborne and, by adjusting the ratio of the minor to total flow, the concentration of coarse particles can be increased by a factor of five or more. Recently, Sioutas et al. (1994) developed virtual impactors separating fine from ultrafine ambient particles. These impactors utilize slit-shaped acceleration and collection nozzles, operate at flows as high as 1000 liters/minute, and have a cut point of 0.1 μm.

Cyclones. Cyclones are devices that, similarly to impactors, utilize particle inertia to separate particles above a given size from the air sample. A typical cyclone is shown in Figure 2.6. The air sample is drawn tangentially near the top. A double vortex is created within the cyclone body. The flow spirals down the outer portion of the chamber, reverses and spirals up the inner core to the exit of the cyclone. Particles that have acquired sufficient

FIGURE   2.6

Schematic Diagram of a Cyclone

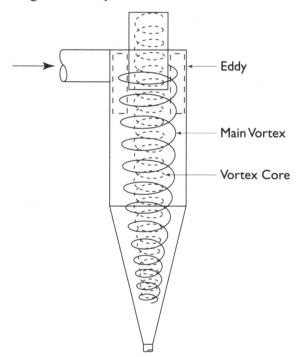

From *Aerosol Measurement* by Lundgren et al., 1976. Reproduced with permission, copyright © University Press of Florida, 1976.

angular momentum due to their inertia, are unable to follow the ascending streamlines and impact on the cyclone walls. Then they either remain on the walls or drop by gravity to the bottom of the cyclone.

Cyclones have been used extensively for collecting dust in industrial processes. They are quite large and operate at flow rates on the order of several cubic meters per second (Hering 1989). Smaller cyclones operated at a few liters per minute have also been popular in aerosol sampling because their penetration characteristics simulate the American Conference of Governmental Industrial Hygienists (ACGIH) respirable mass criteria (Lippmann 1989). Such cyclones are typically used upstream of a filter to remove non-respirable particles, so that the material collected on the filter is representative of the dose to the deeper lung.

Cyclones have several advantages over other inertial classifiers, such as impactors. They are easy to operate, they are not subject to particle bounce, hence do not require special coating for the walls of their chamber (Hering 1989). Their main disadvantage lies in the lack of a theory that describes their performance. Unlike the case of impactors, flow in cyclones is three-dimensional, thus not easily modeled. The dependence of the cutpoint on the flow rate is typically given by an equation in the form (Chan and Lippmann 1977):

$$D_{50} = K Q^n \qquad (2\text{-}2)$$

where D_{50} is the 50% cutpoint, Q is the flow rate, n and K are empirical constants which depend on the design and dimensions of the cyclone. Summaries of theories on the performance of cyclones are given by Chan and Lippmann (1977), and Dirgo and Leith (1985).

Flow pulsation caused by diaphragm pumps can also be a source of sampling errors in cyclones, since it affects the cutpoint. This problem is especially severe in small personal cyclones and has been shown to degrade the cyclone's cutpoint (Saltzman 1984). In addition, the surface of a cyclone can be a sink for reactive gases. Appel et al. (1988) found nitric acid losses as high as 70% on cyclones used as preselective inlets upstream a gaseous collection device (such as denuders, see next paragraph).

Impactor/denuder/filter pack systems. During the last decade, particle sampling systems containing diffusion denuders have been used in a variety of atmospheric monitoring studies (Durham et al. 1978, Ferm 1979, Shaw et al. 1979, Forrest et al. 1982, Braman et al. 1982, and Koutrakis et al. 1988a). In these studies, glass or metallic tubes are coated with an appropriate substance to selectively collect the different gases while allowing other gases and particles to penetrate. Particles are subsequently collected on filter media. Using this sampling technique, particles and gases are separated during sampling, thus sampling artifacts may be minimized. An annular denuder system is shown in Figure 2.7 (Koutrakis et al. 1988).

The principle of operation for diffusion denuders is that gases diffuse to the walls much faster than particles. Consequently, it is possible to trap virtually all of a given type of pollutant gas while a negligible fraction of particles are collected on the denuder walls. Different coating materials can be used to trap different gases. Sodium carbonate (Na_2CO_3), sodium hydroxide (NaOH), and potassium hydroxide (KOH) have been extensively used as a coating substrate because they very efficiently collect acidic gases such as HNO_3, HCl, HNO_2, SO_2, HCOOH, and CH_3COOH (Forrest et al. 1982, Koutrakis et al. 1988, Koutrakis et al. 1993, Lawrence and Koutrakis 1994). Citric acid has been used to collect basic gases such as NH_3 (Koutrakis et al. 1993). Most of the coating substrates are first mixed with glycerol, then dissolved in water or methanol, and subsequently applied to the surfaces of the denuder. The denuders are dried immediately after coating using clean air (Koutrakis et al. 1988).

The denuder/filter pack technology has made possible a number of field and laboratory studies which have enhanced our understanding of the physical chemistry of inorganic atmospheric pollutants. Such systems are cost effective because they allow simultaneous sampling of gases and particles using the same pumping system, which can be the most expensive part of the sampling unit. Moreover, the use of a denuder is necessary to prevent reactions between gases and previously collected particles on the filter media. For example, a significant portion of particulate strong acidity can be neutralized on the Teflon filter by ambient ammonia. Therefore, a citric acid-coated denuder is used upstream from the filter to remove ammonia from the air sample. In addition, either a cyclone (Appel et al. 1988), or a plate impactor (Koutrakis et al. 1990) is placed upstream from the denuder/filter pack to remove coarse alkaline particles. These devices have cutpoints at about 2.5 μm.

Analysis of the Collected Atmospheric Aerosols

Regardless of the type of integrated sampler used for measuring atmospheric particles, the procedure for chemical analysis is generally the same. The collection media (filters, impaction plates) may be weighed to determine the mass concentration of ambient particles, and then subsequently may be analyzed to determine the chemical composition of the particles.

FIGURE 2.7

The Harvard/EPA Annular Denuder Sampler (HEADS)

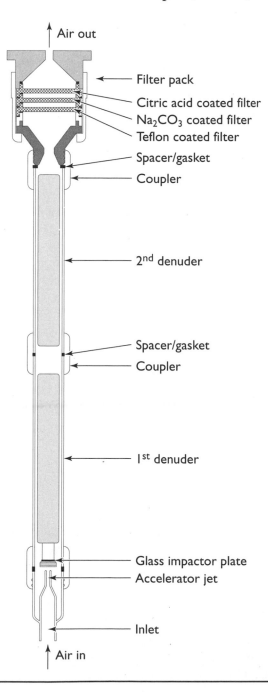

Weighing is typically done before and after sampling with a sensitive microbalance under controlled humidity and temperature conditions.

As discussed previously, ambient particles consist of inorganic elements and ions, including trace metals, as well as graphitic (elemental) carbon and a variety of organic compounds. Below we present some of the most standard types of chemical analysis for determining the chemical properties of ambient particles.

Elemental analysis

The following are the most commonly used techniques for determining the elemental composition of ambient particles.

X-Ray Fluorescence Analysis (XRF). This method has been used for non-destructive elemental analysis of ambient aerosols (Stevens et al. 1978). The sample is irradiated with monochromatic X-Rays. Following excitation, each element in the sample emits characteristic X-Rays which identify the element, and the intensity is used to quantify the concentration of the measured element. Elements lighter than aluminum (Al) are difficult to detect because of their low fluorescent yields and particularly because of the strong absorption of fluorescent X-Rays by the substrate on which they are collected.

Proton-Induced X-Ray Emission (PIXE). This technique is a non-destructive, multi-elemental procedure in which protons excite the atoms of a sample, and the characteristic emitted X-Rays are used to identify and quantify different elements in the sample (Johansson et al. 1975). PIXE is capable of measuring smaller quantities of particulate matter, although it has the same limitations with XRF for light elements. Due to its cost, PIXE is used less frequently than XRF.

Neutron Activation Analysis (NAA). In this method, the sample is bombarded with neutrons, and the radioactivity induced is subsequently measured. Either beta or gamma radiation can be used, but gamma is used more often due to the discrete emission wavelengths which can be used for elemental identification. Depending on the species to be measured, irradiation may last from few seconds to four hours. Limitations of this method include the fact that elements such as sulfur (S), lead (Pb), and cadmium (Cd) cannot be determined by NAA, as well as that NAA is more expensive per sample than XRF and PIXE. NAA has the advantage of higher sensitivity compared to XRF and PIXE, a fact that makes it attractive for sampling trace elements found in extremely low concentrations.

Atomic Absorption (AA). This method is a standard analytical tool for trace metals. The metals are extracted into solution and subsequently vaporized in a flame. A light beam with a wavelength matching the absorption wavelength of the metal of interest passes through the vaporized sample. The light attenuated by the sample is then measured and the amount of the metal present is determined using Beer's law. Atomic absorption has the advantage of being able to measure elements such as cadmium (Cd), lead (Pb), zinc (Zn), and magnesium (Mg). A major drawback, however, is that it cannot be used to detect sulfur. In addition, AA is time-consuming because the collected particles need to be extracted from the filter prior to being analyzed.

Inorganic ions

Inorganic ions, such as sulfate (SO_4^{2-}), ammonium (NH_4^+), and nitrate (NO_3^-), are major constituents of ambient particulate matter and their concentrations are typically measured using ion chromatography. To determine the concentrations of inorganic and organic ions (sulfate, nitrate, ammonium, formate, and acetate), as well as the amount of atmospheric strong acidity (H^+), the filters and the substrates are extracted using ultra-pure water.

One aliquot of the extracted solution is analyzed by ion chromatography coupled with a conductivity detector to determine particulate anion concentrations (NO_3^-, SO_4^{2-} and NH_4^+). To overcome the high conductivity of the eluant, which would overwhelm the sulfate and nitrate signals, the solution passes through a suppression column that contains a strong acid resin; the carbonate is converted to CO_2+H_2O which has a low conductivity, while nitrate and sulfate are converted to their acids (which are highly conductive). This makes it possible to detect the inorganic ions against the suppressed eluant background (Mulik et al. 1976). A second aliquot may be tested for NH_4^+ by ion chromatography, using appropriate separator and suppressor columns.

Another aliquot of the extracted filters and impactor substrates can be analyzed by a pH-meter with a semi-microelectrode to determine aerosol strong acidity, H^+ (Koutrakis et al. 1988). This method uses an electrode in which a potential is developed across a porous glass tube (electrode tip) in the presence of H^+. The magnitude of the potential is logarithmically related to the H^+ concentration, which is the measure of the strong acidity of the collected particles.

Carbon analysis

Carbon is one of the most abundant constituents of ambient particles. It can be present as elemental carbon (EC), which is non-volatile, and as organic carbon (OC), which is volatile. Quartz fiber filters are used as a collection medium because they have a low carbon content and are chemically inert. Carbon analysis is based on the sequential volatilization of organic and elemental carbon followed by oxidation of carbon to CO_2.

A typical analysis is made using a modified Dohrman DC-50 organic analyzer (Huntzicker et al. 1982). Organic carbon is measured by pyrolyzing the samples to CO_2 at 650°C in a helium atmosphere and subsequent reduction of the products to methane over a nickel/hydrogen catalyst bed (Figure 2.8). The generated methane is then measured using a flame ionization detector (FID). After the analysis of organic carbon, elemental carbon is volatilized and oxidized using a 2% oxygen, 98% helium atmosphere at 850°C, converted to methane, and measured with the FID.

Although thermal analysis is a fast and simple method to determine organic and elemental carbon, during the initial heating process elemental carbon can be formed from organic carbon, leading to significant errors. In an attempt to avoid this problem, another method is to digest

FIGURE   2.8

Schematic Diagram of One Type of Thermal Analyzer for Organic and Elemental Carbon

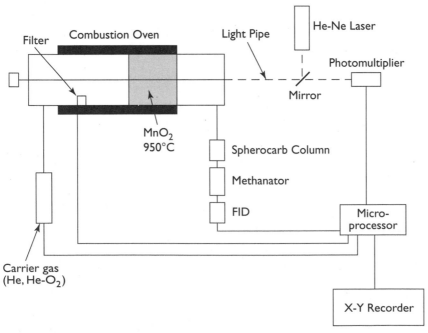

the sample in a strongly oxidizing solution to remove organics and measure the remaining carbon on the filter. Organic carbon is determined as the difference between the total carbon on the filter before and after digestion. However, since some elemental carbon may be removed during digestion (Cadle et al. 1983), this alternate method may not be a significant improvement over thermal analysis.

An improved EC/OC sampler, involving a parallel plate denuder followed by a filter pack, has been developed by the Electric Power Research Institute (EPRI, Palo Alto, CA), and the AeroVironment (Monrovia, CA). This sampler consists of a cyclone that removes particles larger than 2.5 μm from the sample, strips of quartz filter paper in a denuder to remove vapor phase organic carbon, and two back-to-back pre-fired quartz filters to collect particulate EC/OC. The purpose of the secondary filter is to capture particulate phase organic carbon volatilized from the primary filter during sampling. The sampling flow rate is 85 liters/minute (Fitz 1990). Samples are maintained at 0°C during pre- and post-exposure storage and shipping.

Optical methods have also been used to detect continuously graphitic carbon alone (Lin et al. 1973). Light transmitted through a filter that has collected carbonaceous particles is compared to that transmitted through a clean filter to determine the concentration of elemental carbon. The Aethalometer (Model AE-9, Magee Scientific Inc., Berkeley, CA) is an example of a device based on optical methods to determine a surrogate of elemental carbon, called "black" carbon (BC). Light is attenuated by particles collected on a pre-fired quartz filter. The light source is an incandescent bulb with an effective wavelength of 820 nm. An empirically determined factor is used to convert data from this instrument (BC concentration) to EC concentration (Hansen 1984). The performance of this instrument has been tested in field studies and it was found to agree well with independent measurements of EC concentrations (Hansen 1990).

Cooper et al. (1981) converted carbon to CO_2 and then, using a low-background proportional counter, measured the ^{14}C to total carbon ratio. This ratio indicates the fraction of particulate carbon produced by fossil fuel versus that by "modern" sources, such as combustion of vegetation or wood. Fossil fuels contain virtually no ^{14}C, while modern sources present a ^{14}C/total carbon approximately equal to that in the atmosphere.

Organic compounds

The study of organic compounds is necessary in order to identify the sources releasing mostly carbonaceous particles (for example, diesel engines, cars, home heaters, etc). Because of their carcinogenic nature, polycyclic aromatic hydrocarbons (PAHs) have been studied more extensively than any other organic compound. Their sampling and analysis is a difficult chemical problem, because they are partitioned in both gas and particulate phases and their collection is susceptible to sampling artifacts. Analysis of PAHs is typically carried out with high-performance liquid chromatography or thermal separation with a mass spectrometer. The first technique separates the different PAHs, whereas the second determines their mass. Extraction of the sample with an appropriate solvent can separate the organics into acid, base, and neutral fractions, as well as polar and non-polar fractions. Each fraction can be then analyzed by gas chromatographic mass spectrometry (GC-MS) to identify and measure individual organic compounds.

Schueltzle et al. (1975), and Cronn et al. (1977) used high-resolution mass spectrometry to analyze ambient particles. Particle samples were heated to sequentially volatilize various compounds into the source region of the mass spectrometer. Both temperature at which a compound vaporizes, as well as the mass spectrum are characteristic of a particular compound and used for identification. PAHs can be good pollution source tracers. For example, pyrene, fluoranthene, phenanthene are related to emissions from diesel engines, and coronine to gasoline (Gordon et al. 1984).

Crystals. Atmospheric studies have used X-Ray Diffraction (XRD) patterns for the analysis of various crystalline materials to identify particle sources. The greatest obstacle to applying this method to aerosols is low recovery of the particles from the collection medium. Few studies reported successful recovery of crystalline particulate matter from collection media (Brosset 1978, Biggins and Harrison 1979). In the Biggins and Harrison study the particulate matter was collected by an Anderson Impactor modified so that all particulate matter below 2.1 µm would be collected on a single stage. Sampling lasted for a week to allow collection of sufficient material. The collection medium, which was a glass fiber filter paper, was ultrasonicated into aromatic-free n-hexane for 30 minutes and subsequently filtered onto a 0.22 µm millipore cellulose ester filter. The samples were analyzed by XRD with a Philips XDC700 Guiner camera using totally monochromatized Cu radiation.

A similar study, using Teflon filters, was reported by Stevens (1984). Table 2.3 lists minerals that were measured in particle samples collected in four U.S. cities and their chemical composition.

TABLE 2.3

Minerals Commonly Present in Ambient Particles That Can Be Measured by X-ray Diffraction Methodology

Mineral Name	Composition
Biotite	$K_2MgFe_3(FeAl)Al_3Si_3)O_2.(OH)_3$
Muscovite	$KAl_2(AlSi_3O_{10})(OH)_2$
Gypsum	$CaSO_4.2H_2O$
Kalonite	$(FeAl)_4Si_4O_{10}(OH)_8$
Calcite	$CaCO_3$
Plagioclase	$0.55\ [NaAlSi_3O_8] + 0.45\ [CaAl_2Si_2O_8]$
Dolomite	$CaMg(CO_3)_2$
Hematite	Fe_2O_3
Magnetite	$FeO.F_2O_3$
Anglesite	$PbSO_4$
Mascagnite	$(NH_4)_2SO_4$
Thenardite	Na_2SO_4
Sodaniter	$NaNO_3$

Source: Stevens, 1984

Microorganisms

The term "microorganisms" include viruses, bacteria, fungi (e.g., yeasts and molds) and spores of the latter two groups. Spores are clusters of particles from the fruiting body of a fungus or a resistent dormant structure that some bacteria produce to survive adverse conditions (Burge and Solomon 1987). The difficulty in sampling viable microorganisms arises from the fact that they are sensitive to exposure to oxygen, to extreme temperatures, and to humidity while airborne. Thus, although methods for collecting microbial aerosols are similar to those for collecting any other type of airborne particles, the procedures for analysis are very different. Identification of microorganisms can require that collected cells or spores be allowed to multiply to observable numbers. Typically, particles can be collected on semisolid nutrient agar, which is then placed in an incubator to promote cell growth. Particles can also be collected onto filters or in a liquid and transferred to a nutrient agar for growth and possible isolation of bacteria and fungi. Also direct lifting from surfaces can be used to identify microorganisms optically with a microscope or via subsequent culturing.

The literature on sampling airborne microorganisms is quite extensive. Some excellent literature reviews were done by Burge et al. (1987) and

Chatigny et al. (1989). In general, there are two types of efficiencies that need to be considered when sampling airborne microorganisms: 1) the efficiency of the sampler (e.g., the ratio of particles retained by particles entering the sampler), and; 2) the efficiency with which the viability of the microorganism is preserved (recovery). Filters are more efficient collectors of smaller particles, but viable recovery is lower than from an impactor or an impinger. Therefore, there is not a standard sampling method, and the choice of apparatus depends on the viability of microorganism to be analyzed.

Typical liquid media for collecting viruses, bacteria, and fungi include distilled water, physiological saline, phosphate buffered saline, and peptone water. Semisolid media include tryptic soy agar, blood agar, nutrient agar, and heart infusion agar (Chatigny et al. 1989). Nutritionally rich formulas, such as tryptic soy agar for bacteria, and malt extract agar for fungi, are more effective than one that permits differentiation of the collected organisms by selectively promoting or inhibiting growth. Microorganisms can also be detected by staining cells collected on filters (Palmgren et al. 1986), or by assaying the total protein content of the sample as an indicator of biological material. DNA probes and monoclonal antibody labels are rapidly advancing techniques that are being used for microorganism detection.

Summary

Atmospheric aerosols can be generated either through natural or anthropogenic sources. They can also be classified into primary and secondary aerosols, depending on whether they are directly emitted in the atmosphere, or they are generated through gas-to-particle conversion processes. Ambient particles range from 0.01–100 μm. The particle size range from 0.01 to 0.1 μm is known as the ultrafine mode, containing most (in numbers) of the ambient particles. The accumulation, or fine mode consists of particles in the size range 0.1–2.5 μm. Particles in this size range have long residence times in the atmosphere, and can be transported over long ranges. The important chemical constituents of fine particles are sulfate, nitrate, and ammonium ion; organics; and a variety of trace metals. Finally, particles larger than 2.5 μm are known as coarse particles. They are produced by mechanical processes. They are removed from the atmosphere through gravitational settling, although some are returned to the atmosphere through resuspension by the wind.

Sampling of atmospheric particles is a complicated task. Their are two main sampling strategies, depending on the information that is sought.

Direct-reading instruments provide instantaneous information on the concentration and size distribution of aerosols. According to the principle of their operation, these instruments have been placed into four broad categories: optical, electrical, resonance oscillation, and beta attenuation. Direct-reading instruments, however, do not provide detailed information on the chemical composition of particles, which can be obtained by using integrated samplers.

Integrated sampling methods include filters, impactors (inertial or virtual), cyclones, and diffusion denuders followed by filters. The advantages and shortcomings of each of these methods have been discussed. In general, there is no optimum method, and the choice of the sampling technique depends on the type of compound to be sampled and the type of analysis to be performed. Filters are the simplest method, and can be used with non-volatile compounds. However, when sampling compounds that exist in both particle and gas phases, impactors and denuders should be preferred.

Before any chemical analysis is performed, the total collected aerosol mass may be measured. Subsequently, the elemental composition of particles can be determined. Elemental composition of particles can be determined by X-Ray diffraction, particle-induced X-Ray emission, neutron activation, and atomic absorption. Inorganic ions, such as sulfate, nitrate, and ammonium, can be determined using ion chromatography. Particle acidity is measured by determining the concentration of hydrogen ions using a pH-electrode. Organic and elemental carbon are determined using thermal methods. Volatile organic carbon vaporizes first, whereas elemental carbon is oxidized at the highest temperatures. Elemental carbon can be also measured through light attenuation techniques (aethalometry). Various crystalline materials are detected using X-Ray diffraction. Microorganisms are collected on a semisolid nutrient agar, or in liquid media, and then placed in an environment that promotes their growth prior to their counting.

3

Emissions, Dispersion, and Concentration of Particles

John Spengler and Richard Wilson

Emission and Composition of Particles

To examine the role of outdoor PM_{10} and $PM_{2.5}$ on respiratory health effects one must consider the variability in space and time of the composition of the particles and of their sources. The U.S. air quality standards set by the EPA recognized the importance of measuring size fractionated particle mass when it established the PM_{10} standards. Some argue that this distinction between PM_{10} and TSP is insufficient. Both the production and the physiology suggest that finer distinctions are useful.

Particle size is expressed in terms of its aerodynamic diameter, defined as the diameter of a unit density sphere that has the same settling velocity (Hinds 1982). Typically the mass of PM exists in the atmosphere in a bimodal size range, with peaks occurring between 0.1–1.0 µm, and 2–10 µm ranges (Whitby and Sverdrup 1980). The sources contributing to these two mass ranges (fine and coarse particle modes, respectively) may differ, which in turn are reflected in their chemical composition. The idealized mass distribution of atmospheric aerosols discussed in Chapter 2 described the compostion of particulate matter in the lower atmosphere, and various sampling methods. Prior to discussing the relationship among outdoor, indoor and personal exposures to particles in Chapter 4, it is useful to know something about the spatial distributions of particle concentrations in the U.S. and elsewhere. It is important to distinguish particle mass and composition by size. Two decades ago, Whitby and Cantrell (1975) presented a stylized representation of particle size distribution in a "typical" atmosphere, along with important sources and mechanisms responsible for particle removal. Figure 3.1 shows the idealized size distribution of the aerosols (by volume). For instance, the origin of particles

FIGURE 3.1

Schematic of Deposition and Coagulation of Particles

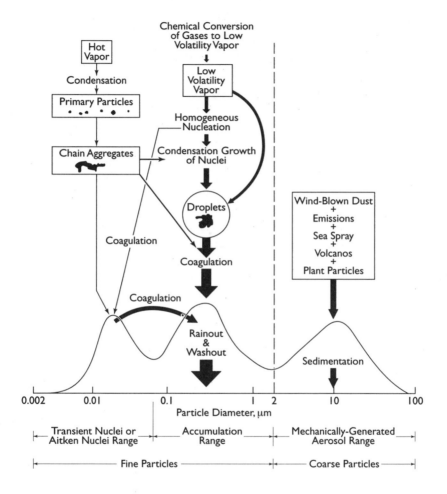

Based on Whitby and Sverdrup (1980)

in the fine or respirable range is generally from high temperature processes such as fuel combustion or metallurgical operations emitting vapors of high boiling liquids, which tend to condense on particles with large surface areas i.e. fine particles. Such emissions may exist initially in particle sizes less than 0.1 μm, but rapidly accumulate into the 0.1–1.0 μm range. Tobacco smoke and particles generated by atmospheric reactions (e.g. photochemical smog) ultimately exist in this size range. The components of aerosols in the 0.1–1.0 μm tend to be sulfates, acids, metal salts, and carbon. Markers for combustion-related fossil fuel sources include sulfur and certain metals such as vanadium, nickel, and selenium. Table 3.1 contrasts fine and coarse mode particles in terms of their composition, sources, expected lifetimes, and travel distances (persistence).

Inhalation of Particles

The size, shape, density and reactivity of particles determine how they will be transported and react in the human respiratory tract. Target sites within the respiratory tract vary with the aerodynamic size of particles as well as other factors. This can be seen by examining the variation of respiratory penetration and retention with particle size shown in Table 3.2 to the composition of atmospheric particles as shown in Figure 3.1. Most of the particles greater than 10 μm in diameter and about 60–80% of particles of 5–10 μm are trapped in the nasopharyngeal region. Larger particles are subject to inertial and centrifugal focus. Very small particles (<0.1μm) penetrate and deposit deeper in the lungs by diffusional forces. Air is moving slowly and distances are short. The lungs are least efficient at retaining the particle sizes that accumulate in the atmosphere (ICRP 1966). A prediction (ICRP 1966) of the deposition of particles of various sizes on various parts on the respiratory tract is shown in Figure 3.2.

T A B L E   3 . 1

Comparison of Fine Versus Coarse Mode Particles

	Fine Mode	Coarse Mode
Composed of:	Sulfate, $SO^=_4$; Nitrate, NO^-_3; Ammonium, NH^+_4; Hydrogen ion, H^+; Elemental carbon, C; Organic compounds; PNA; Metals, Pb, Cd, V, Ni, Cu, Zn; Particle-bound water; Biogenic organics.	Resuspended dusts, soil dust, street dust. Coal and oil fly ash. Metal oxides of Si, Al, Mg, Ti, Fe. $CaCO_3$, NaCl, sea salt, pollen, mold spores, plant parts.
Sources:	Combustion of coal, oil, gasoline, diesel, wood. Atmospheric transformation products of NO_x, SO_2, and organics including biogenic organics, e.g., terpenes. High temperature processes, smelters, steel mills, etc.	Resuspension of soil tracked onto roads and streets. Suspension from disturbed soil, e.g., farming, mining. Resuspension of industrial dusts. Construction, coal and oil combustion, ocean spray.
Lifetimes:	Days to weeks	Minutes to hours
Travel Distance:	100s to 1000s of kilometers	1 to 10s of kilometers

Source: Wilson et al., 1995; Draft Particle Criteria Document, Chapter 3 (1995)

FIGURE   3.2

Regional Deposition Predictions Based on the Model Proposed by the International Comission on Radiological Protection Task Group on Lung Dynamics

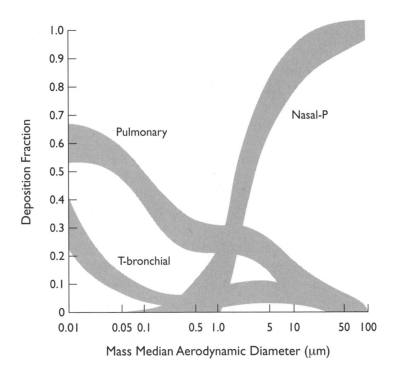

Each of the shaded areas (envelopes) indicates the variable deposition for a given mass median (aerodynamic) diameter in each compartment when the distribution parameter σ_g varies from 1.2 to 4.5 and the tidal volume is 1,450 ml. From ICRP (1966).

Nevertheless particles smaller than 2.5 μm are breathed deeply into the lungs and therefore expected to present a risk greater than a comparable mass concentration of larger particles. These particles circumvent many of the respiratory system's defense mechanisms, such as cilia, and are capable of delivering relatively high concentrations of potentially harmful substances, often causing severe damage at the cellular level (Amman et al. 1986). Li, Lin, and Jeng (1993) demonstrated that 2 μm particles are generally caught in nose cilia before reaching the lungs, but mouth breathing can facilitate the deposition of these particles that reach the lungs. These facts lend biological plausibility to the observations in Chapters 6

T A B L E   3 . 2

Respiratory Penetration vs. Particle Size

- 11 μm and up particles do not penetrate
- 7–11 μm and up particles penetrate nasal passages
- 4.7–7 μm particles penetrate pharynx
- 3.3–4.7 μm particles penetrate trachea and primary bronchi
- 2.1–3.3 μm particles penetrate secondary bronchi
- 1.1–2.1 μm particles penetrate terminal bronchi
- 0.65–1.1 μm particles penetrate bronchioli
- 0.43–0.65 μm particles penetrate alveoli

Note: The US EPA's National Ambient Air Quality Standard (NAAQS) defines "inhalable particles" as those with aerodynamic diameters less than 10 μm (PM_{10}).

---

and 7 that the observed effects on health of particle are associated with fine particles rather than course particles. Mechanisms of toxicity in animals are discussed in detail in Chapter 5 and mechanisms in people are discussed in Chapter 8.

Emissions Inventory

Various attempts have been made to inventory pollution emissions in the U.S. In Table 3.3 we show the estimates of 1990 emissions made by Pechin and Associates (1994,1996). These authors present an illusory indication of accuracy by presenting many significant figures. We have modified their original table to round the numbers off to one or two significant figures which is as accurate as we believe the numbers to be.

The final column adds together the $PM_{2.5}$ fraction and the sulfur and nitrogen oxides which will probably become particulates. These, if totally converted, which is likely for sulfur oxides which are emitted from tall stacks and less likely for nitrogen oxides that are emitted close to the ground, outnumber the original $PM_{2.5}$ by 4 to 1. As shown in these estimates almost half of fine particle emissions originate as sulfur from coal burning.

Nitrogen oxides come from fuel burning as the nitrogen and oxygen in the air are combined by the reaction with or without a catalyst. At the high temperature of a flame the equilibrium pushes the reaction to the right, producing nitrogen oxide. If the gases cool slowly the reaction proceeds again from right to left and the nitrogen oxide breaks up. If the cooling is rapid, there is no time for the break up again, and the NO persists. At the present time, stationary sources and motor vehicles produce approximately equal amounts of nitrates. In principle the nitrogen oxides, and hence the nitrates, can be eliminated completely by feeding pure oxygen to the flame,

T A B L E   3 . 3
1990 U.S. Particulate Emissions

Source Category	PM$_{2.5}$	PM$_{10}$	Precursors SO$_2$	NO$_x$	PM$_{2.5}$ + secondaries
Electric Utility Coal	100,000	270,000	15,000,000	6,700,000	22,000,000
ditto Oil and Gas	6,000	11,000	600,000	800,000	1,400,000
Fuel use—industrial	180,000	250,000	3,000,000	3,000,000	6,500,000
Fuel use—commercial	15,000	35,000	600,000	700,000	1,200,000
Residential wood	500,000	500,000	9,000	66,000	570,000
Chemical Manufacturing	40,000	60,000	400,000	400,000	850,000
Metals Processing	100,000	140,000	900,000	80,000	1,000,000
Petroleum industry	20,000	30,000	400,000	100,000	500,000
Other industry	250,000	400,000	400,000	300,000	1,000,000
Storage and Transport	30,000	60,000	5,000	2,000	30,000
Waste disposal/recycle	200,000	230,000	40,000	80,000	300,000
Highway engines	300,000	350,000	500,000	7,000,000	8,000,000
Non road engines	200,000	220,000	300,000	3,000,000	3,500,000
Agricultural burning	1,000,000	1,200,000	7,000	200,000	1,200,000
Wind erosion	800,000	5,000,000	0	0	800,000
Road dust	3,000,000	17,000,000	0	0	3,000,000
Construction	1,600,000	8,000,000	0	0	1,600,000
Agricultural tilling	1,400,000	7,000,000	0	0	1,400,000
Total	10,000,000	42,000,000	22,000,000	23,000,000	55,000,000

Data from Pechin et al. 1994, 1996

or by controlling the flames carefully, or catalytic recombination. Adding ammonia to the combustion gases reduces the emissions of NO and NO$_2$ by accelerating convection to ammonium nitrate.

Here we have *not* listed Total Suspended Particulates (TSP). But an inspection of Table 3.3 shows that road and other dusts will be the major contributor to TSP.

The U.S. EPA reports that PM$_{10}$ emissions have decreased slightly since the mid 1980s. Reductions have been noted for the fuel combustion category and in wood combustion. Where there has been aggressive public education, restrictions and improved stove design particle emissions from domestic burning of wood has been reduced. While reduction in some categories of particulate emissions and for SO$_2$ and NO$_2$ precursors have been substantial, PM$_{10}$ emissions from vehicles have increased. Between 1983 to 1992 a 50% increase in the Highway Vehicle category was calculated. Until transportation related ozone compliance strategies are implemented, particle emissions from mobile sources is expected to increase still further.

The contribution of fugitive dust sources to airborne concentrations of PM_{10} can be seen from Table 3.3. These calculations suggest that construction, agriculture, driving on unpaved roads and wind erosion emissions are nearly ten times all other direct PM_{10} emissions combined. These fugitive dust sources are hard to control. The contribution of fugitive dust to the smaller size fraction $PM_{2.5}$ is only three and a half times the other direct contributions and the secondary aerosol formation from SO_2 and NO_2 emissions dominate. Unfortunately for the decade spanning 1990, there has not been much reduction in SO_2 emissions. In fact, the fuel combustion component actually increased somewhat. Effects (if any) of tracking SO_2 emission permits are not expected to be observed until the later half of the 1990s. If the 10 million tons per year reduction in SO_2 that is expected takes place, atmospheric sulfates will decrease and so will the concentrations of $PM_{2.5}$ and to a lesser fractional extent PM_{10}.

Measured Particle Concentrations

In this section we show some concentrations as measured in the U.S. Total suspected particulate (TSP) matter was designated as a national criteria pollutant by the Clean Air Act Amendments of 1970. Until July 1987 TSP was the only widely available measurement of particle air pollution in the U.S. In July 1987 EPA started to use PM_{10} to represent suspended particles in the air. Between 1988 and 1992 some 652 sites nationwide operated to establish trends and determine compliance with the annual (50 μg/m³) and 24 hour (150 μg/m³) NAAQS. Figure 3.3 displays in box-plot format the distribution of annual average PM_{10} concentrations. The boxes show the spatial distribution over the sites. The limits are the 10th and 90th percentiles and the next boxes are the 25th and 75th percentiles. A 17% reduction over this time period is shown. However, there are still many locations in the U.S. that exceed either annual or daily NAAQS. Figure 3.4 shows the locations in the U.S. that are in non-attainment. The box diagram of Figure 3.5 examines the 90th percentile of the 24-hour PM_{10} concentrations for the 799 trend sites. There has been a downward trend (~20%) and decrease in the variance (spread of distribution between sites).

Concentrations monitored at ambient locations do not fully indicate the extent of actual exposures to PM_{10}. The next chapter describes the relationship of ambient levels to indoor concentrations and personal expo-

FIGURE   3.3

Boxplot Comparisons of Trends in Annual Mean PM_{10} Concentrations at 652 Sites, 1988–1992

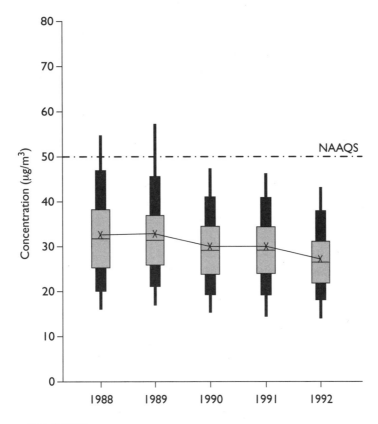

Source: EPA (1995b)

sures. As a first approximation the "population at risk" can be estimated by taking county air pollution measurements and the number living in those counties exceeding standards. EPA defines preadolescents ($\leq$13 years old), elderly ($\geq$65 years old) and those with pre-existing respiratory conditions such as asthma, emphysema and chronic obstructive pulmonary disease. Table 3.4 estimates the population at risk in the U.S. Obviously, not all these people experience ambient PM_{10} levels over the standards.

In contrast to TSP which can very rapidly change from place to place, PM_{10} concentrations only vary over larger distances of several kilometers. Many locations with elevated concentrations are near industrial sources or in drier and dustier regions. Individuals with severe respiratory prob-

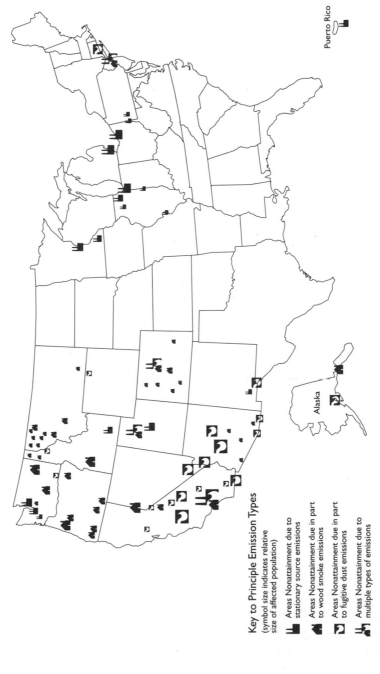

Areas Designated "Non-Attachment" for Particulates (PM₁₀)

Key to Principle Emission Types
(symbol size indicates relative
size of affected population)

Areas Nonattainment due to
stationary source emissions

Areas Nonattainment due in part
to wood smoke emissions

Areas Nonattainment due in part
to fugitive dust emissions

Areas Nonattainment due to
multiple types of emissions

Source: EPA (1995b)

FIGURE 3.5

Distribution of 90th Percentile of the 24-hour PM_{10} Concentrations Across 799 Monitoring Sites

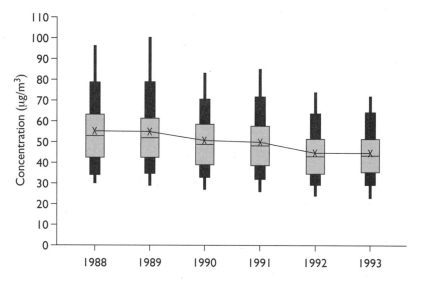

Boxes show the range of the data.
Source: EPA (1995b)

lems are less active, spend more time indoors and use air conditioning and air cleaners more than the normal population. So the population estimated in Table 3.4 should be considered as an upper bound estimate for the population heavily exposed to PM_{10}. If the true hazard of particulate exposure is disproportionately in the fine fraction then knowing the relationship between $PM_{2.5}$ and PM_{10} is important. Also relevant is the fraction of $PM_{2.5}$ penetration into homes and buildings which is discussed in Chapter 4.

The chemical composition of the measured PM_{10} and fine particles differs from region to region. The pie charts of Figure 3.6 show the contribution of different sources of PM_{10}, the fine fraction $PM_{2.5}$, and the coarse fraction $PM_{10}–PM_{2.5}$ in the eastern and western United States. In general, the fine particles in the eastern U.S. are comprised of relatively more sulfate (47 per cent) than the west (15 per cent). The proportion of organic carbon in Western U.S. urban areas is about twice the proportion in Eastern U.S. urban areas. In addition, the majority of western sites tend to have a lower sulfate and a larger nitrate composition. Fine particles, especially sulfates and nitrates also contribute to visibility reduc-

FIGURE 3.6

Contributions of Different Sources of Particulate Matter[a]

Eastern U.S. Urban Areas   **Western U.S. Urban Areas**

PM$_{2.5}$

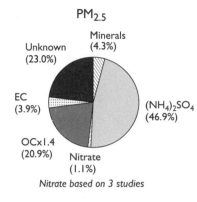

Minerals (4.3%)
Unknown (23.0%)
EC (3.9%)
(NH$_4$)$_2$SO$_4$ (46.9%)
OCx1.4 (20.9%)
Nitrate (1.1%)

Nitrate based on 3 studies

PM$_{2.5}$

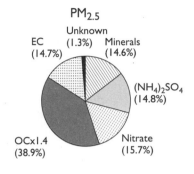

Unknown (1.3%)
EC (14.7%)
Minerals (14.6%)
(NH$_4$)$_2$SO$_4$ (14.8%)
OCx1.4 (38.9%)
Nitrate (15.7%)

Coarse Fraction

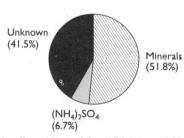

Unknown (41.5%)
Minerals (51.8%)
(NH$_4$)$_2$SO$_4$ (6.7%)

Insufficient Nitrate, OC, and EC data available

Coarse Fraction

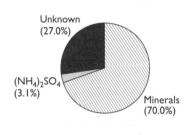

Unknown (27.0%)
(NH$_4$)$_2$SO$_4$ (3.1%)
Minerals (70.0%)

Insufficient Nitrate, OC, and EC data available

PM$_{10}$

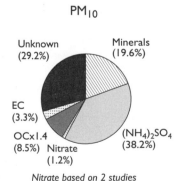

Unknown (29.2%)
Minerals (19.6%)
EC (3.3%)
OCx1.4 (8.5%)
Nitrate (1.2%)
(NH$_4$)$_2$SO$_4$ (38.2%)

Nitrate based on 2 studies

PM$_{10}$

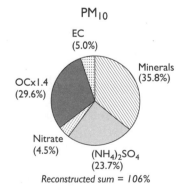

EC (5.0%)
Minerals (35.8%)
OCx1.4 (29.6%)
Nitrate (4.5%)
(NH$_4$)$_2$SO$_4$ (23.7%)

Reconstructed sum = 106%

[a]Sulfate as ammonium sulfate; Carbon as organic carbon multiplied by 1.4 for oxidized species; Elemental carbon; Nitrate as NO$_3^-$;Minerals assume stable forms found in earth crustal materials

Source: EPA (1995b)

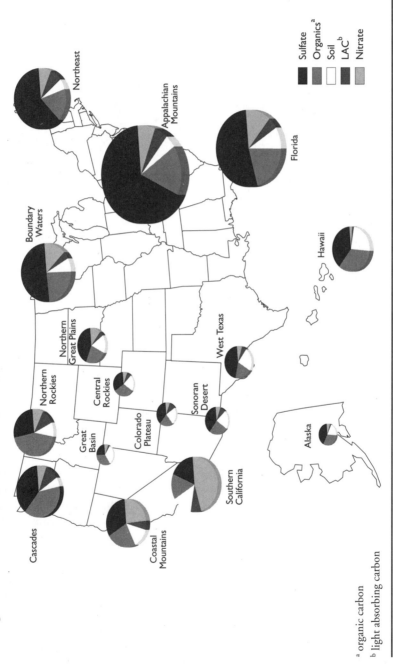

FIGURE 3.7
Average Annual Extinction, from EPA (1993)

a organic carbon
b light absorbing carbon

TABLE 3.4

Estimated Number and Percentage of Total U.S. Population and At-Risk[a] Subgroups Residing in Counties with Particulate Air Pollution (PM$_{10}$) Exceeding Daily Levels of 155 µg/m³ and 55 µg/m³ in 1992

Population at Risk	PM$_{10}$ levels ≥ 155 µg/m³		PM$_{10}$ levels ≥ 55 µg/m³	
	Number	%[d]	Number	%[d]
Total Population	22,894,856	9.1	114,671,632	45.5
Preadolescent Children (aged 13 years and under)	4,931,408	9.5	23,794,139	46.0
Elderly (aged 65 years and over)	2,649,477	8.3	14,010,297	44.1
Persons under 18 years with asthma	386,220	9.5	1,878,848	45.9
Persons over 18 years and over with asthma	697,444	9.1	3,528,475	46.2
Persons with chronic obstructive pulmonary disease[e]	1,243,407	9.1	6,263,409	46.0

Source: Vigliarolo et al. 1994

[a] Population-at-risk estimates should not be added to form totals. These categories are not mutually exclusive.

[b] PM$_{10}$ of ≥155 µg/m³ is the federal "exceedance" definition; PM$_{10}$ ≥55 µg/m³ is the California "exceedance" standard.

[c] The PM$_{10}$ level of the county does not imply responsibility for the disease status of its population.

[d] Of the total population in the category, the proportion of each population subgroup potentially exposed.

[e] Includes chronic bronchitis and emphysema.

tion and atmospheric discoloration. The map of Figure 3.7 shows the contributions of various particle fractions to visibility reduction in the U.S. The size of each pie shows the total extinction in the region and the pie itself shows the contribution of each component.

The presence of sulfates, in terms of the spatial distribution of ambient PM, merits further discussion. Power plants, the largest sources of SO$_2$ (which ultimately forms sulfates), are located principally east of the Mississippi River in the eastern U.S. and Canada. Their emissions tend to be released from tall stacks leading to regional formation of sulfates. Sulfate particles almost entirely in the submicron size range, however, are observed to display less spatial variation at a community level (Suh et al. 1995, Özkaynak et al. 1996a). Personal monitoring studies show that personal and outdoor sulfate levels are well correlated (Suh et al. 1993, Özkaynak et al. 1996a). However, when it comes to acidic sulfur compounds there is considerable inter and intrapersonal variation. Activity patterns and neutralization by ammonia are contributing factors (Suh et al. 1992). This illustrates exactly the conundrum that we face. For some components and size fractions, ambient particulate concentrations measured at a few locations in a community may well represent the population, while for other components there is poor correlation between outdoor and personal concentrations as is discussed in more detail in the next chapter.

Air Dispersion

General

The transport and dispersion of pollutants emitted high into the atmosphere can prevent the buildup of potentially hazardous concentrations. The first mitigation step, therefore, was to establish an appropriate separation between polluting sources and humans breathing near the ground. This was accomplished horizontally by zoning and vertically by building tall chimney stacks. The natural dilution occurring in the atmosphere seemed a sufficient pollution control strategy for several centuries. Unfortunately, this is not now the case. In urban areas as well as rural towns, sources and receptors are close. Often there is insufficient separation, for example, between an airport and its neighbors, or the traffic and a pedestrian walkway. Even where sources have been placed further away, terrain and meteorology can adversely affect dilution.

Now there are many such sources emitting into a common air mass. The pollutants can be transformed into other chemical species that remain in the atmosphere for days. Carried along in the mass of air, they can be transported back to populated areas, affecting millions of people.

In order to understand air-pollution health effects and controls, and assign them to individual emission sources, we must discuss atmospheric dispersion processes numerically. We rely on mathematical estimations of air pollution concentrations to design control strategies, set new source performance standards, prescribe chimney heights, test source compliance with ambient air quality standards, and prevent significant deterioration of air quality. There are numerous other applications of air pollution dispersion modeling. These include the modeling of photochemical reactions and transport, visibility impacts, and regional transformation and transport of sulfates.

In this section we discuss in an elementary way the important models used in air pollution studies. They are usually variations of three types.

■ A simple proportional model can be used to estimate the amount of emission reductions needed to achieve a proportional reduction in ambient concentrations. This type of modeling was applied extensively in the 1960s and early 1970s as local and state air pollution control agencies devised fuel sulfur regulations and transportation control plans.

■ At the opposite end of the scale are the numerical simulation models using derivations of the Navier-Stokes equation for fluid flow. This model requires specification of boundary as well as initial conditions across the spatial array of interest. Concentrations are estimated by a stepwise finite differentiation scheme. This type of model has been extensively used in photochemical modeling, where the intermediate concentrations of a number of reactive pollutants are needed.

■ The third and most widely used formulation of atmospheric dispersion is based upon the idea that the turbulent structure of the lower atmosphere having a Gaussian or normal statistical distribution. That is, the eddies or turbulence in the air (Taylor 1922) act on the emitted pollution in such a way that the concentrations will be distributed normally around a peak center-line concentration.

Gaussian plume or Lagrangian models are used for primary pollutants, such as particulate matter, NO_2, SO_2, and air toxics. More complex models are needed to address and include chemical transformations, such as the link between NO_x emissions and ozone concentrations and SO_2 to sulphate concentrations. Primary pollutants are classified as those that do not undergo chemical transformation between the time they are discharged and inhaled or ingested by the receptor. It must be remembered that for areas with complex topology and complex meteorology, such as urban and coastal settings, Gaussian models may have to be adjusted. Mathematical functions describing the decay can be added to the formulae to handle losses and chemical reactions.

Gaussian models are usually reliable for short distances of 10 km or less, but are in fact, commonly applied to distances up to 50–80 km, and for these cases such as radionuclide emissions where a population dose is sufficient to assess the impact on the regional population.

For regional modelling, most analysts prefer Eulerian grid or Lagrangian trajectory models. Examples are the Harwell Trajectory Model and the European Monitoring and Evaluation Program (MEP). These models correctly track air masses from place to place while correctly taking into account continuity criteria.

Dispersion from a single chimney stack: the Gaussian Plume model

The basic formula for the spread of pollution from a stationary source was the Gaussian Plume model developed by Sutton (1932). The concentration of a pollutant is described by the product of two empirical Gaussian distributions, one for vertical spread including "reflection" from the ground and one for horizontal spread perpendicular to the prevailing wind direction (each varying with distance along the plume, x). The plume width parameters which are input into the model, are based on empirical correlations and take into account relevant meteorological conditions.

$$C = \frac{Q}{2\pi u \sigma_y \sigma_z} \exp\left(-\frac{y^2}{2\sigma_z^2} \right) \left\{ \exp\left(-\frac{(z-h)^2}{2\sigma_z^2} \right) + \exp\left(-\frac{(z+h)^2}{2\sigma_z^2} \right) \right\} \quad (3\text{-}1)$$

C = the concentration of pollutant in quantity per unit volume (g/m^3).

Q = the quantity emitted per unit time (in g/s) by a chimney stack considered to be at the origin of coordinates. The coordinate axes are chosen as shown in Figure 3.8 so that the wind travels with velocity u along the x axis.

The z axis is vertical and xy plane ($z = 0$) is the ground.

σ_y and σ_z are the standard deviations of the normal distribution densities of the dispersion. They depend upon travel distance as the plume spreads with time.

h = the height of the plume, not simply the stack height because buoyant exhaust gases usually make the plume rise even after leaving the stack, although adverse meteorologic conditions can cause downwash.

This equation is included here because of its historical importance. It, together with a categorizing of weather conditions by Pasquill (1961, 1962), was used to aid in much of the air pollution reduction since 1945. A useful categorizing of the parameters σ_y and σ_z and modifications can be found in Turner (1972, 1979). This equation can easily be used to describe several elementary features, such as the existence of a skip distance such that pollutant concentrations are low until a distance where $\sigma_z \geq h$, and for larger distances the concentration is independent of stack height.

FIGURE 3.8

Schematic of Gaussian Plume Model

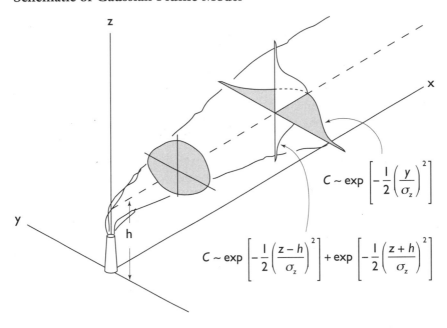

$$C \sim \exp\left[-\frac{1}{2}\left(\frac{y}{\sigma_z}\right)^2\right]$$

$$C \sim \exp\left[-\frac{1}{2}\left(\frac{z-h}{\sigma_z}\right)^2\right] + \exp\left[-\frac{1}{2}\left(\frac{z+h}{\sigma_z}\right)^2\right]$$

Long-range transport and dispersion

When considering dispersion of pollutants beyond 30 km, the Gaussian model described in the preceding section is less appropriate, because it does not describe the movement of the air mass into which the pollution is diffusing or penetrating by convection. As already mentioned, additional factors must be considered.

- Deposition rate of SO_2 (cm/sec)

- Deposition rate of SO_4 (cm/sec)

- Transformation (conversion) rate for SO_2 to SO_4 (%/hr)

- Transformation rate for NO_x

- Diurnal charges of the mixing height in the atmosphere

- Primary sulfate (% of emitted SO_2)

For example SO_2-to-sulfate conversion rates have been reported to range from 0.2 to 3 percent per hour. Even if the conversion rate is as low as 0.5 percent per hour, it is high enough to produce a great deal of sulfate from an elevated source of SO_2. Gases and particles from a 200 m high stack will travel 20,000 m at a wind speed of 5m/s for about an hour before the spreading plume strikes the ground. It will take longer before half of the plume has come in contact with the ground. Then, based on these assumptions considerable conversion will have taken place.

There are two competing processes removing SO_2 from the plume, dry deposition at the ground and conversion to the sulfate particulates in the air. Today less than one seventh of the SO_2 released into the air over the U.S. is from small stacks less than 120 feet (36.5m) in height. Discharge of emissions (at heights of a few hundred meters or more enhances SO_2 to sulfate conversion and long range transport because the atmosphere is more stable, and winds are stronger, than closer to the ground.

The models that can be used to estimate sulfate, nitrate (and ozone) concentrations include (Systems Applications Incorporated (1987,1989):

- Harwell Trajectory Model (HTM) for regional transport and chemistry of sulphur and nitrogen emissions

- Windrose Trajectory Model (similar to HTM)

- European Monitoring and Evaluation Program (EMEP) transfer matrix for acid deposition

- Sector average Limited Mixing Mesoscale Model (SLIM3)

The models that can be used to estimate ozone concentrations include:

- Ozone Isopleth Plotting Mechanism (OZIPM-4) (Environmental Protection Agency (1987, 1989)

- Mapping Area-Wide Predictions of Ozone (MAP-O_3) (McIlvaine (1994)

- KAMM-DRAIS model of the University of Karlsruhe.

Figure 3.9, already used in Wilson et al. (1980), depicts the modeled annual mean sulfate concentrations over the U.S. based on emissions from major coal-burning facilities. The pattern of high sulfate particle concentrations in the eastern third of the U.S. reflects both the distribution of sources and the climate. In 1996 a similar situation prevails. About 80% of all SO_2 emissions come from within the 31 states bordering on or located east of the Mississippi. In spring and summer the prevailing winds are from the southwest on much of the eastern U.S.

FIGURE 3.9

Predicted Annual Sulfate Concentrations Modified from the Brookhaven Long-Distance Transport Model

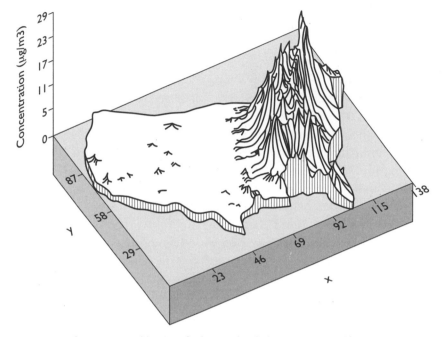

Emissions are from major coal-burning facilities and include area sources. Sulfate concentrations (in μg/m³) are proportional to altitude and spatially averaged over 32 x 32-km grids (x, y). (From Wilson, Colome, Spengler and Wilson 1980)

Global averages

For very small particles, large distances, and long term spatial and time averages, the problem simplifies again. Pollutants will spread widely. It is easy to see that a removal mechanism must be postulated or the calculated effects will increase without limit. If the particles are trapped between the ground and an inversion layer without removal, the concentration averaged over all possible wind directions will fall as $1/r$. The population within an area between a radius r and $r + dr$ from the source is $2\pi r\, dr$. If the effect on an individual in the population is proportional to concentration the integrated effect at a radius r is proportional to the product of these two factors and is independent of r. As we further integrate over all r the upper limit of the integration will be determined by some removal mechanism to obtain a finite answer.

For a particulate which has no chemical action in the atmosphere, deposition is a function of particle size. All particles are driven downwards by turbulent diffusion which is enhanced for large particles by g ravitational setting. For gravitational settling Stokes' law (equation 2-1) applies, and the deposition velocity varies as the square of the diameter. For small particles, less than 0.1 μm, the deposition velocity is determined by Brownian motion. There is a characteristic minimum of the plot of deposition versus particle size at about 0.5 μm. Below 2.5 μm the deposition velocity is about 0.1 cm/sec. Measured values are characteristically between 0.1 and 1 cm/sec.

If the pollutants are trapped in a 2000 m layer of the atmosphere, the residence time for a deposition velocity of 0.1 cm/sec becomes 200 days. With a typical stable wind of 7 m/sec, the pollutants can travel 13,000 km! It is likely that the most important removal mechanism for these particles is then wet deposition by rainfall. The concentrations will vary is the inverse of the average rainfall frequency.

This will then give an average over wide regions determined primarily by the total emissions in the region, and the frequency of the depositing rainfall. Then one may make a simple didactic model that *all* the SO_2 converts to sulfates before hitting the ground; and that the removal process is rainfall every few weeks.

Predictions and tests of long range transport

In a demonstration that conversion of gases to particulates actually occurs, McMurry et al. (1981) (Figure 3.10) showed how the particle size distribution changes at a distance from a power plant. The coarse fraction of PM_{10} decreases with distance. The fraction (relative amount) of the fine particles (around 0.3 μm) increase, largely by conversion of SO_2 to sulfates and NO_x to nitrates.

The first extensive test of long-range transport was performed for the Office of European Cooperation and Development (OECD 1977). They carried out two set sof tests. In one set, individual pollutant masses were followed. One, for example was seen to pick up pollution in the Ukraine, travel over Europe to Spain, out over the Bay of Biscay, and turn eastwards again over northern Scotland to Scandinavia. Another test carried out by OECD was to confirm that their model, an early Lagrangian model, could predict *average* particulate concentrations over many diverse monitoring stations.

Prediction of behavior in extreme accident situations is very important because in these situations any threshold for health effects can be exceeded

FIGURE 3.10

Volume-Size Distribution Taken in the Midwestern United States Near the Cumberland Power Plant in Tennessee

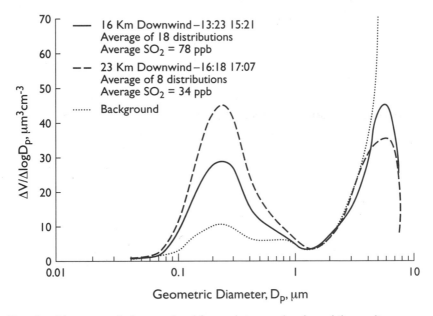

Note that the coarse mode descreased and fine mode increased as the mobile sampling van moved downwind farther from urban influence but allowing more time for reaction as the power plant plume mixed with background air, and SO$_2$ was converted to sulfate and NO$_x$ to nitrate.
Source: McMurry et al. (1981)

and strong measures such as evacuation may be needed. However, even the best modelling now available cannot predict the detailed behavior of individual air masses. The ARAC model which at the time was the least available, did not describe a major feature of the radioactivity deposition after the Chernobyl accident: the deposition 80 miles NE of the plant near Gomel (Belarus) and Briansk (Russia). It was mostly in this region that children ingested or inhaled radioactive iodine and developed thyroid cancers. The deposition occurred during a rainfall on Sunday evening April 27th, 36 hours after the accident. The model did not include rainfall, and rainfall was not added in "by hand." It is not certain that U.S. scientists and authorities were aware of it and of its importance. The U.S. ARAC model was very successful in showing that most of the initial plume went westwards, but some, at a higher altitude, went eastwards toward Japan and Asia (Dickens and Sullivan, 1986; Gutiksen, Sullivan and Harvey, 1986).

The Kuwait oil fires, starting in February 1991 and continuing through October 1991 offered a magnificent opportunity to test these models. The main feature of the weather pattern in that period was the prevailing wind from NW to SE, which, most of the time, blew the smoke away from the city of Kuwait and down the gulf where it was obvious to the naked eye 300 km away in Bahrain and Dharhan. The heat from the fires caused the smoke to rise and collect above a temperature inversion layer at about 1,000 m. Airplanes flew into the plume and recorded concentrations of pollutants, (which agreed well with calculations [Sullivan et al. 1994]), but the all-important concentration of pollutants on the ground depended upon the more subtle penetration of pollutants across the inversion layer. The *average* behavior of the plume was reasonably well described. However, some individual deviations, in which for example air masses turned westward over Riyadh in Saudi Arabia, were not well described even after the event (WMO 1992).

These failures of the predictions of the models are not usually considered to be failures of the models themselves, but a statement that the information that is input to the models, wind directions, rainfall etc., is often, perhaps usually, inadequate. However, global averages over both space and time are more likely to be reliable. Therefore we must depend for guidance on the global averages described above.

Summary

The characterizations of particles by size is important both because of their mechanisms of production, coagulation and depositions in the environment, but also because of the way in which they are deposited and retained in the human lung and respiratory tract.

In the atmosphere sulfur oxides and nitrogen oxides are often connected to fine particles. The emissions inventory of particle sources has only recently been characterized by size. The most important contributors to the fine particle (PM 2.5) concentrations are electic utility (particularly coal) industry, industrial fuel use and mobile (highway) engines.

Ultimately, dispersion models can be used as part of an estimate of health damage expected from single or multiple sources of pollution by calculating population exposures. The critical component that is needed is an appropriate model for the health damage to be used with the dispersion model.

4

The Role of Outdoor Particulate Matter in Assessing Total Human Exposure

Haluk Özkaynak and John Spengler

Introduction

Over the centuries, people have been concerned about air pollution, but primarily in occupational settings (mines and factories) and outdoors in urban areas. The concentrations of pollutants at these locations often far exceeded concentrations indoors. But since the 1952 London air pollution episode, the reduction in outdoor particle pollution in the U.S., Japan and Western Europe (OECD countries) has been considerable. At the end of the 1970s peak concentrations were one tenth of earlier values and averages were also reduced. It has also been argued that people spend over 80% of the time indoors, where exposures to outdoor air pollution is greatly reduced. These two facts together suggested (to some scientists) that the associations between air pollution and mortality found by Lave and Seskin (1977) could not be real.

Exposures to outdoor particles have traditionally been considered the most important component of total personal exposures. Over the last decade, however, the composition and concentration of ambient or (i.e. outdoor) particulate matter (PM) has changed substantially. Air pollution control efforts have led to significant reduction in the deposition of settleable dust and soiling across most industrialized and urban areas of the U.S. In general, the effectiveness of particulate emission control equipment is based on the efficiency of particulate removal, measured as a reduction in mass rate of emissions. Since large particles account for the bulk of the emission mass, these industrial control efforts had little effect on the concentrations of particles in the fine or respirable size range. Moreover, reliance on tall stacks has facilitated the dispersion of fine particles and their precursor gases over extended regions in the United

States. For example, emissions of sulfur oxides and selenium from power plants in Ohio River Valley, has been linked with higher concentrations of sulfates in the eastern United States (Wilson et al. 1980, Thurston and Spengler 1985). Furthermore, increases in local emissions of particulates, such as from wood burning or diesel vehicles in some locations have increased the ambient concentrations of respirable particles and have led to reduced visibility.

Communities long ago recognized the health consequences of exposure to pollutants in ambient air. Air pollution control programs were directed towards reducing the emissions of outdoor particulates with the expectation of major air quality and health benefits to be derived from such reductions. However, over the last decade or so, total exposure assessment studies for CO (Akland et al. 1985), VOCs (Wallace 1987, et al. 1991), pesticides (EPA 1990), and PM (Wallace 1996, Özkaynak et al. 1996) began providing a more complete understanding of the relative contribution of outdoor pollutants to total personal exposures. It is now well known that for many air pollutants, even those where the major sources are outdoors, there is substantial variability in population exposures. Among the factors contributing to variability in personal exposures are the impact of indoor sources, the time-activity profile of the individuals in the population (i.e., the amount of time spent in various microenvironments) and spatial variability in ambient concentrations. As research has progressed it has become clear that in many instances, ambient monitoring at fixed locations does not adequately or accurately reflect the exposure of the human population (Ott et al. 1988, Spengler and Soczek 1984, Brauer et al. 1989). In particular, for many pollutants, exposures encountered while indoors or in the individuals immediate vicinity are found to be substantial. Therefore, the ideal epidemiologic analysis of mortality or morbidity records would utilize total personal exposures to particulates and not just community-averaged outdoor PM levels in the statistical investigation of exposure-response relationships. Answering the question of how well outdoor levels of PM define actual human exposure and the associated health consequences requires insight into the processes leading to total exposures. It is necessary to discuss the original size distribution outdoors, dispersion in the ambient air, penetration across the building envelope, and exposure to the human respiratory tract. Human beings come in contact with pollutants of outdoor origin in many settings (microenvironments) including: ambient locations, indoors at home, at work or in school, in transit while commuting or riding in a car or a bus.

The fundamental assumption of most air pollution epidemiologic studies and compliance monitoring, for that matter, has been that concentration of outdoor particulate matter (PM) serves as a surrogate for personal exposure as well as dosage. However, many animal and human health studies have shown that the health effects resulting from PM exposure are a function of the mass, size and composition of particles deposited in the different regions of the respiratory tract over a specified time interval. The amount of the potential dose depends on the concentration inhaled, ventilation rate, and fractional deposition, which in turn is influenced by factors such as breathing mode, anatomical structure of airways, and alterations attributable to lung dysfunction. Since all people do not have identical ventilation rates or deposition patterns, the potential dosage distribution cannot be linearly scaled to the personal exposure distribution (Adams, 1993). If outdoor particulates contribute to exposures in a predictable fashion and are relatively substantial then it may be possible to rely on measurements of outdoor PM concentrations in epidemiologic investigations of health effects of exposures to airborne particulates. In this chapter we examine the relevant findings from recent field monitoring programs in the context of epidemiologic models to examine this hypothesis.

The previous chapter (3) provided a brief description of the nature of airborne particulates, in terms of sources, composition, and spatial/temporal distribution in the U.S. In this chapter the primary question to be resolved is the relationships between ambient PM concentrations and personal exposures. This will depend in part, on the penetration of fine particles into indoors where we spend most of our lives. Several studies have contributed to the understanding of indoor/outdoor PM correlations and how this is related to total human exposures. For completeness, numerous studies are cited which examine sources, exposures, and indoor/outdoor concentrations. Finally, the critical question about using outdoor pollution measurements to represent personal exposures in epidemiologic studies is discussed.

Studies of Indoor, Outdoor and Personal PM Concentrations

The recognition that actual exposures to PM and other pollutants might be quite different than depicted by outdoor samplers became the mantra for those advocating better understanding of the indoor/outdoor (I/O) relationships. Biersteker et al. (1965) conducted the first major study of I/O air pollutant relationships in the Netherlands. The particulate measurement methods were specifically designed for PM ("smoke") and SO_2. Rather than the recent techniques discussed in Chapter 2 for measuring PM concentrations, these historic measurements were based on the reflectance of the collected particle deposit, and subsequently converted to mass concentration measurements. The results of this pioneering work, however, demonstrated that indoor concentrations of PM were quite different from outdoor concentrations, and the realization that indoor sources (such as improperly vented heating systems) could have a profound effect on indoor air quality.

Subsequently, numerous studies measured I/O relationships for PM using the Hi-Volume sampling technique for TSP. Yocom et al. (1971) measured PM in homes and office buildings in the Hartford, Connecticut area using two methods. One technique utilized a miniaturized version of a high-volume sampler, which collected particles up to 30 μm size range. In the second method, light absorbance of the PM deposit was converted to a Coefficient of Haze (COH per 1000 lineal feet of air sampled). This device sampled particles in the range of 5–10 μm and indicated that there was more penetration of outdoor particles in this size range than TSP.

Lioy et al. (1985) conducted a brief indoor/outdoor study of respirable PM ($PM_{2.5}$) in and near a home in New Jersey. The $PM_{2.5}$ samples were extracted with three different organic solvents of increasing polarity. The outdoor samples were collected on the roof of a nearby building. The I/O ratios for the solvent extractable particulate matter were greater than one, and suggested significant penetration of this type of material, results which were in a range similar to Yocom et al. (1971).

Dockery and Spengler (1981a) studied the indoor-outdoor relationships of respirable sulfates and particles in 68 homes in six U.S. cities. A conservation of mass model was derived describing indoor concentrations in terms of outdoor concentrations, infiltration and indoor sources. The measured data were analyzed to identify important building characteristics and to quantify their effect. The mean infiltration rate of outdoor fine particulates was found to be approximately 70%. Cigarette smoking was found to be the dominant indoor source of respirable particulates. In addition to ambient contribution, increased indoor concentrations of sulfates were found to be associated with smoking and also with gas stoves.

Dockery and Spengler (1981b) conducted a study of personal exposure to $PM_{3.5}$ and sulfates in Watertown, MA, one of the cities in the Six Cities Study. The authors clearly demonstrated that the results from fixed indoor samplers in the homes of subjects were better predictors of total exposure than fixed outdoor samplers located throughout the community being studied. As part of the research effort, a model was developed based on time-weighted activity patterns of each subject from which total exposures could be calculated. Table 4.1, based on 37 observations, shows how well indoor and outdoor measurements and the activity pattern model predicted total exposure. These results indicate that the indoor measurement of sulfate, a pollutant of primarily outdoor origin, is a good predictor of personal exposure. In the case of $PM_{3.5}$, a pollutant with both indoor (smoking) and outdoor sources, there was greater scatter in the data than for sulfate, and neither of the measurement modes nor the model were particularly good predictors of personal exposure. However, indoor measurements were better than those outdoors alone in predicting personal exposure to $PM_{3.5}$.

As part of the Six Cities Study, Spengler et al. (1981) took measurements of $PM_{2.5}$ indoors at homes in three communities for two weeks in winter and again in the summer. The difference in mean concentrations between smoking and non-smoking households was greater in winter than in summer in all cities. Similar results were observed by Quackenboss (1991), who studied effects in spring and fall seasons as well. As the focus shifted to pollutant composition and season-dependent sources, Santanam et al. (1990) reported on another aspect of the same study—source apportionment using Principal Components Analysis. Cigarette smoking, wood-burning, sulfur-related sources, and auto-related sources were among the key contributors to $PM_{2.5}$ mass indoors during the seasons studied. Non-smoking homes in the two cities had indoor mean $PM_{2.5}$ concentrations very close to outdoor mean values. In two related studies, Sheldon et al. (1989) and Leaderer et al. (1990) evaluated the effect of kerosene heaters, gas stoves, wood stoves, or fireplaces, and cigarette smoking on indoor concentrations of combustion products. These stud-

TABLE 4 . 1

Fraction of the "Between Subject" Variance Explained by Outdoor Means, Time-Weighted Exposure Model, and Indoor Means as Estimators of Personal Exposure (37 Observations)

	Outdoor Measurement	Time-Weighted Model	Indoor Measurement
Sulfate	0.654	0.765	0.728
$PM_{3.5}$	0.479	0.570	0.514

Source: Dockery and Spengler 1981b.

ies confirmed that smoking was the single most powerful source of indoor fine particles—regardless of season.

Suh et al. (1992, 1993) conducted two studies examining personal exposures. The first study measured personal exposures and I/O relationships of acidic aerosols and gases in Uniontown, Pennsylvania, and compared these data with measurements at a central outdoor monitoring station. The results suggested that personal sulfate models based on outdoor measurement, time activity data, and home air conditioning status may be used to estimate exposures to children in other, similar communities (Suh et al., 1992). A subsequent study using similar techniques as in the 1992 study, was carried out in State College, Pennsylvania (Suh et al., 1993). The micro environmental exposure model developed in the Uniontown study was refined and applied to the State College data. Personal exposures to sulfates and hydrogen ions (H+) showed considerable variability among subjects. Nevertheless, the sulfate and H+ models with the highest accuracy and precision were based on outdoor and indoor concentrations, activity patterns, and a correction factor for H+. The exposure model predictions for sulfate were better than those for H+, results which were attributed to greater variability in H+ and NH_3 concentrations. Indoor concentrations of NH_3 exceeded those outdoors, while indoor measurements of HNO_3 and H+ were lower than those outdoors because of the neutralizing effect of NH_3.

Özkaynak, et al. (1995, 1996b) described the first major field study carried out in the fall of 1990 under the PTEAM program. This study was carried out on a probability-based sample of 178 non-smoking individuals aged 10 or older residing in Riverside, CA, a site subject to wide swings in outdoor PM concentrations. Each study participant carried PM_{10} personal exposure monitor (PEM) for two consecutive time periods, each of approximately 12-hour duration (nominally 7 P.M. to 7 A.M. and 7 A.M. to 7 P.M.). No personal sampling was done for $PM_{2.5}$. At the conclusion of each personal monitoring period, each subject was interviewed to obtain data on various activities including those that might affect exposure to PM (proximity to smokers, cooking, gardening, etc.). Simultaneous with the personal monitoring, PM_{10} and $PM_{2.5}$ samples were collected indoors by a stationary indoor monitor (SIM) in the main living area, and outdoors by an identical stationary ambient monitor (SAM) at each home. Measurements using several PM sampling methods were made at a fixed central site during the duration of the program generating 96 consecutive 12-hour samples. The samplers at the central site consisted of a PEM, a SAM, two Wedding high-volume PM_{10} samplers, and two Anderson dichotomous samplers. All filters were subjected to gravimetric analysis and elemental analysis by X-ray Fluorescence (XFR).

Based on an analysis of the data from this program the authors concluded that personal exposure to PM_{10} for non-smokers was high in comparison with outdoor ambient concentrations. Personal exposures to PM_{10} tended to be greater than either indoor or outdoor concentrations during the active 12 hours of the day, but that difference was much less evident during the quiescent period. Analysis supports the concept that personal activities, particularly those spent away from home, increased the likelihood that the volunteer encountered locations where PM_{10} concentrations were higher. Exposure to environmental tobacco smoke (ETS) is such an example, but there were other unidentified sources.

While personal activities and exposures (e.g., smoking and cooking) are responsible for some of this difference, Özkaynak et al. (1996b), propose that other factors may come into play such as modification of sampling rate for personal monitors because of the motion imparted on the sampling system by the subjects as they go about their normal activities, and the "personal cloud" of the subjects that include such personal emanations as skin flakes and lint from clothing.

The earth crustal elements Cu, Al, Si and Fe tend to be higher outdoors than indoors. This is supported by the rather low correlations between indoor and outdoor levels. These same related elements are also higher for the daytime personal sample lending further support to the idea that the subjects were being exposed to more larger particles outdoors and away from home.

Elemental sulfur which is predominantly in the fine particle fraction tends to be uniformly distributed in the outdoor air mass and reflects the day to day changes in S content of the air mass. Also, the indoor-outdoor correlation of S across all homes was highly significant (>0.9). This indicated that the fine fraction of the aerosol mass penetrates readily to the indoor environment.

Leaderer, et al. (1994) performed an indoor-outdoor sampling program for $PM_{2.5}$ in 394 homes in Suffolk and Onondaga Counties, NY in late winter and early spring of 1986. Homes were selected based on various indoor activities and the presence of potential sources of PM (e.g., smoking, gas stove, wood stove, fireplace, kerosene heater, and humidifier). The collected samples were weighted to produce a weight concentration of aerosol and were subjected to elemental analysis by X-ray fluorescence. The data showed that gas stoves and humidifiers do not contribute to indoor aerosol mass and elemental concentrations. Smoking was the single most important source influencing indoor aerosol concentrations. In this work the presence and use of a wood stove did not appear to contribute significantly to indoor concentrations of aerosol. The indoor concentration of S, except for homes with operating kerosene heaters, showed that this element is primarily of outdoor origin, and I/O ratios were in range that agreed well with other workers. As has been found by other workers, lead is an element of outdoor origin. Indoor and outdoor concentrations of crustal elements such as Si, Fe, and Mn were similar for all homes indicating indoor sources since lower concentrations would be expected. As noted before, soil tracked into the house and becoming re-entrained is a likely indoor source.

Koutrakis et al. (1992) preformed a source apportionment of New York particle data set. The results were consistent with the PTEAM study findings in that smoking influenced indoor $PM_{2.5}$ concentrations and sulfur was related to outdoor sources.

Predicting Personal and Indoor PM Exposures

In practice, all air pollution epidemiology done to date has related human health outcomes to ambient concentration rather than personal exposures or dosage. Exposures studies have been used to identify the modifiers of exposure such as passive cigarette smoke, gas cooking, kerosene heating, air conditioning, or outdoor activity time. In the absence of direct personal monitoring data researchers have relied upon models to predict personal and indoor PM concentrations using available data on outdoor PM concentrations, human time-activity data and physical building parameters that affect penetration of outdoor pollutants indoors.

A variety of physical and statistical modeling methods have been developed for predicting exposures to gases and particles (See for example, Duan 1982, Ott 1985, Spengler and Soczek 1984, Lioy 1990, Ryan 1991). In this framework total exposure E_t is modeled as a sum of exposures encountered in various microenvironments (E_i).

Predicting personal PM exposures

Daily personal exposures (E_i) are computed as the sum time-activity weighted microenvironmental exposures:

$$E_i = \sum_{j=i}^{m} E_{ij} = \sum_{j=1}^{m} f_{ij} \bullet C_{ij} \qquad (4\text{-}1)$$

where, E_{ij} = exposure to individual i in microenvironment j ($\mu g/m^3$), f_{ij} = the fraction of time spend by person i in microenvironment j during the 24-hour prediction period, C_{ij} = the average PM_{10} concentration ($\mu g/m^3$) in microenvironment j when individual i is present and m is the number of microenvironments considered in the model. Accuracy and the precision of the microenvironmental exposure models depend on the number of different microenvironments that are needed to capture most of the variations in the concentrations affecting exposures. Clearly, if activities or concentrations of PM do not vary much across different locations that individuals visit over the course of a day, fewer number of microenvironments are sufficient to model personal exposures. In general, five principal microenvironments may be included in the $PM_{2.5}$ and PM_{10} exposure models to represent the distinct PM exposure locations/activities. These are:

■ Outdoors

■ Indoors at home during daytime (7:00 A.M.–7:00 P.M.)

■ Indoors at home during nighttime (7:00 P.M.–7:00 A.M.)

■ In transit

■ Indoors not at home

Various $PM_{2.5}$ and PM_{10} exposure scenarios within these micro environments (or submicroenvironments) need to be considered. These may include: a) smoking or ETS exposure indoors and in car; b) cooking at home.

In practice PM_{10} measurements available from ambient air monitoring sites are used to estimate the outdoor particle concentration profiles across a community. Whereas, the indoor residential or at work PM concentrations are estimated using semi-empirical methods that account for penetration of outdoor pollutants indoors and contribution of indoor sources, such as smoking, cooking, vacuuming, etc. to indoor PM levels. Measurements of $PM_{2.5}$ and PM_{10} across different urban areas indicate that $PM_{2.5}$ concentrations are highly correlated between different sites while PM_{10} are correlated less strongly. In Philadelphia, Burton et al. (1996) found correlations near 0.9 to 1 for $PM_{2.5}$ and correlations of around 0.8 for PM_{10} across 7 sites in Philadelphia. Ito et al. (1995) also found correlations around 0.7 to 0.8 among PM_{10} measurements in Chicago and Los Angeles when the distances between pairs of sites were less than 20 miles. In Riverside, CA, PTEAM study correlations between 0.8 to 0.85 were obtained when central site PM_{10} measurements were related to measurements taken outside of the 175 study homes (Özkaynak et al. 1995).

Since most people spend large portions of their time indoors, the indoor air concentrations are also important. A recent nationwide study of time budgets in the U.S. indicates that residents spend 87.2% of their time indoors, 7.2% in transit, and 5.6% outdoors (Robinson and Nelson, 1995). Clearly, indoor environment plays a key role in effecting personal exposures since most of our time during the day is spent either indoors at home or at work or at school. In addition to examining the impacts from particles generated indoors, it is important to understand how concentrations of outdoor particles are attenuated as they infiltrate indoors. Both indoor and outdoor particles contribute to concentrations of indoor PM. The level of protection or attenuation offered by building characteristics can directly influence the resultant exposure to ambient particles such as PM_{10} and $PM_{2.5}$. Building specific parameters such as volume, air exchange rate, filter efficiencies, surface materials, dust loading activity levels, room use patterns as well as cleaning frequency all affect the cumulative particle concentrations. The air exchange rate contributes to dilution of indoor PM source concentrations, such as from smoking or cooking, yet will directly affect the penetration of ambient particles..

Indoor PM concentrations can be modeled using the methodology developed from the PTEAMS study by Özkaynak et al. (1995, 1996b). A semi-empirical physical model which assumes contributions to indoor PM_{10}, from: outdoors, environmental tobacco smoke (ETS), cooking, and other unaccounted indoor sources. The PTEAMS study had measured indoor and outdoor PM_{10} in 175 homes during two consecutive 12-hour periods: daytime (7:00 A.M.–7:00 P.M.) and nighttime (7:00 P.M.–7:00 A.M.). Thus, the indoor PM models estimates separately for the two time periods the contributions of the outdoor and indoor sources of PM_{10}. The general structure of the physical model is given as:

$$C_{in} = \frac{P.a}{a+k} C_{out} + \frac{N_{cig}S_{smk} + T_{cook}S_{cook}}{(a+k)Vt} + \frac{S_{other}}{(a+k)V} \qquad (4\text{-}2)$$

where:

C_{in} = PM_{10} or $PM_{2.5}$ concentration indoors

C_{out} = PM_{10} or $PM_{2.5}$ concentration outdoors

P = Penetration fraction (unitless)

a = air exchange rate (hr^{-1})

k = PM$_{10}$ decay or deposition rate (hr^{-1})

N_{cig} = number of cigarettes

V = house volume (m^3)

T_{cook} = cooking time (hr)

S_{smk} = estimated source strength for cigarette smoking (mg/cig)

S_{cook} = estimated source strength for cooking (mg/hr)

S_{other} = re-suspension or estimated source strength for other indoor sources (mg/hr)

t = sampling period (12 hrs)

Using this physical model formulation and the PTEAMS data Özkaynak et al. (1996b) had estimated the PM$_{10}$ source strengths, removal rate and penetration fraction with the nonlinear estimation technique (NLIN) available on SAS. These parameters (e.g. P, k, etc.) are especially important in estimating the average contribution of outdoor particles to indoor PM concentrations.

Some of the articles in ambient (outdoor) air are able to enter the airspace of an enclosed (indoor) environment. For a given particle, the predominant characteristic determining the probability of penetration is its size. Larger particles may be filtered out or once inside, settle out relatively quickly. Smaller particles can penetrate easily indoors. The penetration factor P represents the ability of a particle to penetrate a building envelope. For inert gases, the expected value of P is 1. For very large particles, whose P-value (in the absence of open windows or doors) would be expected to go to zero as particle size increases. Two recent studies have used different methods to determine the P value for a range of particle sizes. As mentioned above, the PTEAM study (Özkaynak et al., 1996b) statistically determined a value of 1 for PM$_{10}$ and PM$_{2.5}$ penetration into residences using a nonlinear solution of a full mass balance equation, including all indoor sources for 175 homes. Thatcher and Layton (1995) used an experimental technique, directly measuring one instrumented house. They, too, found a P-value of 1 for all the size ranges tested, including 1–3 μm, 3–5 μm, 1–5 μm, 5–10 μm, and 10–25 μm. Thus, the two studies independently arrived at the same conclusion: particles less than 10μm in aerodynamic diameter penetrate building envelopes with the same efficiency as (nonreactive) gases. Although more work may be needed to experimentally validate this finding, the assumption that P equals unity for all size ranges less than 10 μm allows us to estimate of the effect of outdoor air particle concentrations on indoor levels and personal exposures.

Also using, the PTEAM database, Murray and Burmaster (1995) have taken the analysis one step further to calculate the fraction of outdoor air particles found indoors at equilibrium. Based on Equation 4-2 this fraction is equal to $Pa/(a+k)$. As shown in Figure 4.1, at a mean air exchange rate of 0.76hr^{-1}, which is typical of an ordinary residence in the winter time, the fraction of outdoor fine ($d_a < 2.5$ μm) and coarse ($2.5 \leq d_a \leq 10$ μm) are 66% and 43%, respectively. The exact placement will depend on the relative proportions of fine and coarse particles constituting the PM$_{10}$. These results indicate that the contribution of outdoor PM$_{10}$ or PM$_{2.5}$ to indoor (and personal) exposures is sizeable, or about 50%. Moreover, these results also suggest that certain practical mitigation measures (e.g. reducing air exchange rate, installing air conditioning or weatherizing)

FIGURE 4.1

Fraction of Indoor PM From Outdoor Airborne PM, Under Equilibrium Conditions, as a Function of Air Exchange Rate, for Two Different Size Fractions

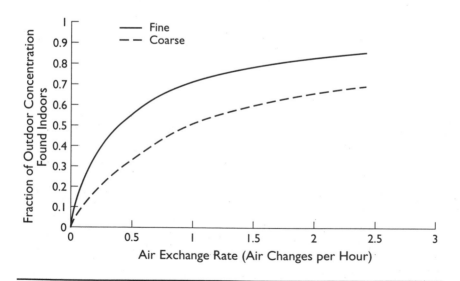

could reduce indoor PM exposures for persons at an increased risk of adverse health effects from outdoor pollution.

The Relationship Between Ambient PM and Personal Exposures

Several studies suggest that ambient concentrations are not correlated with either indoor concentrations, or exposures. Hence, outdoor concentrations cannot serve as a surrogate to determine exposure. For instance, in the Netherlands, Janssen et al. (1995) reported that correlations of personal PM_{10} exposures and ambient PM_{10} were poor ($R^2 = 0.11$ for children; $R^2 = 0.02$ for adults). Similarly, Bahadori et al. (1996) studied personal exposures to PM_{10} and $PM_{2.5}$ in Nashville, Tennessee, and concluded there was a nonsignificant (negative) correlation between personal and ambient monitors.

It has been proposed (Mage and Buckley, 1995; Spengler et al., 1985) that such a discrepancy may be attributable to two factors: human exposure to PM at work and in traffic are only partially accounted for in measurements of I/O PM values, and indoor/outdoor averages reflect periods of low concentrations during which the subject may not be present. In some instances individuals engage in particle generating activities in microenvironments where exposures to PM_{10} might be high but brief. An important example for this situation is exposure to ETS in homes, restaurants or offices in which fine particle concentrations exceed 100 µg/m³ over exposure periods less than 30 minutes (Repace and Lowrey, 1980).

Jannsen et al. (1995) found an explanation for the apparently discrepant results. They pointed out that there is considerable variation between subjects, for example there will be a large difference between those exposed and not exposed to environmental tobacco smoke (ETS). The low correlations observed in other studies were mostly determined by the variation between subjects (e.g. same regression for subjects exposed and not exposed to ETS). They re-examined their $PM_{2.5}$ data, and averaged the daily means. The result, shown in Figure 4.2 suggests a much stronger correlation between the personal measurements and the ambient concentrations.

Similar findings were recently reported by other researchers also. By reanalyzing the Phillipsburg, NJ personal and outdoor PM_{10} data from Lioy et al., 1990, Mage and Buckley (1995) showed that the relationship between personal PM_{10} and outdoor PM_{10} could be dramatically improved if daily averages of personal PM_{10}, instead of individual personal PM_{10} measurements are regressed against the mean outdoor PM_{10} values.

FIGURE 4.2

Comparison of Personal and Ambient Pollution Measures for PM$_{2.5}$

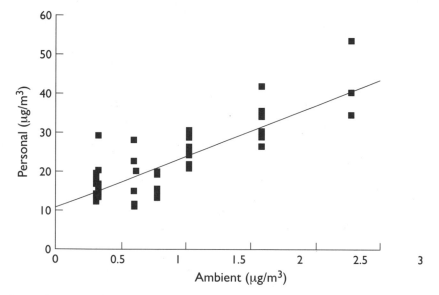

Source: Jannsen et al. (1995),

The predictive power of the models were shown to increase from 0.25 to 0.91 simply by averaging the personal PM$_{10}$ data. Using the same data set Wallace (1996) also showed that when individual longitudinal (consecutive 14 day) regressions on personal exposures of concentrations at the nearest outdoor site are calculated, the ability of the outdoor sites to explain the variance in personal exposures is greatly increased over the cross-sectional regressions. The median R^2 of the 14 individual (longitudinal) regressions was found to be 0.46 compared to the median R^2 of 0.06 found for the 14 daily (cross-sectional) regressions. Essentially the same phenomenon was found by Dockery and Spengler (1981) when they showed that between community exposures to personal sulfates reflected differences in ambient levels.

As in the case of the Mage and Buckley (1995) analysis, a similar improvement in the predictive power of the personal vs. outdoor PM$_{10}$ models were found in further analysis of the Riverside, California PTEAMS personal and outdoor PM$_{10}$ data. Figure 4.3 shows daily individual personal PM$_{10}$ values regressed against the daily outdoor PM$_{10}$ data. The R^2 of the regression model is 0.16 which is not good. In contrast Figure 4.4

FIGURE 4.3

Comparison of *Daily Individual* Personal and Outdoor PM_{10} Concentrations in Riverside, CA (PTEAMS)

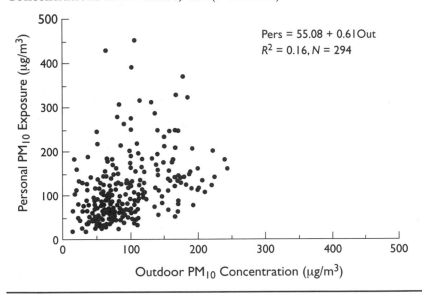

shows the daily *average* personal PM_{10} regressed against the daily average outdoor PM_{10} data. The R^2 of the regression model doubles (i.e. increases from 0.16 to 0.33). These results, and others referred to in Mage and Buckley (1995), suggest that, even though, it is difficult to precisely estimate any given individual's personal PM_{10} exposure on a particular day based on outdoor PM measurements alone, nevertheless, it is still possible to reasonably estimate either community average or individual multi-day personal exposures using the available outdoor PM_{10} measurements. The implications of these findings to epidemiologic studies of particle health effects utilizing outdoor PM data are quite important. We examine this issue further in the next section.

Errors in Using Ambient PM Concentrations in Epidemiologic Studies of Particle Health Effects

Over the past two decades our understanding about the relationship between outdoor and indoor concentrations, and in particular the relationship between outdoor concentrations and personal exposures has been shaped by numerous studies. Obviously, indoor concentrations of particles are a function of both outdoor and indoor sources. However, most epidemiologic studies do not account for the effects of indoor and out-

FIGURE 4.4

Comparison of *Daily Averaged* Personal and Outdoor Concentrations in Riverside, CA (PTEAMS)

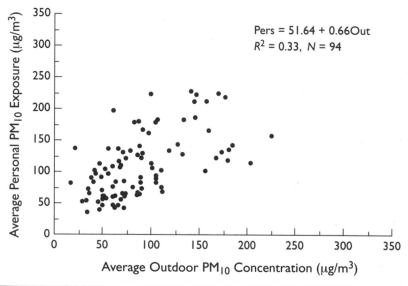

Pers = 51.64 + 0.66Out
$R^2 = 0.33$, $N = 94$

door PM exposures. Mage and Buckley (1995) took a new look at numerous personal exposure studies. By developing aggregate measures of exposures, they observed a relationship between outdoor concentrations and personal exposures. This was apparent when averages rather than individual values of personal PM exposures are correlated with ambient PM concentrations. As discussed earlier these findings were also suggested by the analysis of the extensive PTEAMS PM_{10} data from California where there was substantial day-to-day variation in outdoor PM_{10} concentrations. In retrospect it now seems that the interpretations of earlier indoor and personal exposure studies were influenced by the following conditions:

■ Low outdoor concentrations with little spatial and temporal variations

■ Integrated indoor and outdoor concentrations that could not provide time resolved correlations to activity and location data

■ Reliance on mass concentration rather than chemical and elemental data to discriminate among sources.

Clearly, *on a mass basis* the contribution of outdoor particles to indoor and personal concentrations are not very large if and when the outdoor ambient levels are low. However when outdoor concentrations are high the influence of ambient particles on indoor concentrations can be observed. In contrast, for homes with no smokers, field data and physical modeling show that indoor/outdoor ratios are about 60–70% for $PM_{2.5}$ and about 50% for PM_{10} (Özkaynak et al. 1996b and Wallace 1996). Personal PM_{10} exposures are influenced by outdoor PM_{10}. The data from PTEAMS show that about 60% of outdoor PM_{10} is expected to contribute to personal PM_{10}.

The two critical issues of importance to epidemiology of ambient particle health effects are:

■ the relative toxicity of ambient particles compared to indoor particles, and

■ the error introduced in the statistical analysis of health and pollution data when using ambient PM measurements as a surrogate for personal exposures.

The toxicity of outdoor air pollutants and particles and gases from specific sources continues to be assessed with animal studies. Urban particles with acidic, organic and metal constituents have been linked to a variety of physiologic and pathogenic changes in respiratory responses, inflammation, infection and cardiovascular responses. Less well characterized are indoor sources with the exception of cigarette smoke, and perhaps NO_2 and CO from combustion.

Indoor particles are sometimes generated on a regular basis and sometimes on a less routine basis. Cooking and cigarette smoking might occur daily at regular intervals. But holiday events, visitors, vacuuming, remodeling are not necessarily daily activities. Also, because of home and building operating schedules there can be diurnal, weekly and seasonal cycles of indoor particle generation. Mainly because of meteorological factors, episodes of high ambient pollution also tend to occur, but are not correlated with the generation of indoor particles. Therefore, both longitudinally or cross-sectionally ambient PM concentrations (especially $PM_{2.5}$) might be expected to correlate well with the community-average personal PM concentrations. Because indoor sources are affecting personal exposures differentially across a community, the relative toxicity of ambient vs. indoor particles should not appreciably distort the estimated health effects of ambient particles that are used in some epidemiologic analyses.

The appropriateness of selecting ambient PM concentrations as a suitable exposure metric is often raised in the context of epidemiologic analysis of health effects of particulates (Lipfert and Wyzga, 1995a,b). This alters the errors (uncertainty) of the exposure measures in the regression analysis, which can be addressed statistically. Lipfert and Wyzga (1995a,b) have questioned the validity of epidemiologic air pollution mortality studies on various grounds, including difficulties in model specification, proper accounting of weather effects, uncertain pollution exposure estimates and problems with multicollinearity among different pollutants. Perhaps the most serious criticism they have raised has been in connection with the limitations of using ambient pollutant concentrations instead of actual personal exposures in estimating statistically the magnitude and the strength of association between PM_{10} and health effects. Even though the topic of effects of errors of measurement on multiple correlations have been studied by statisticians for many years, it's application to air pollution epidemiology has been quite recent.

Cochran (1970) has examined the problem of errors in variables and its effects on regression modeling results. In particular, Cochran (1970) calculated the relationship between R^2, the squared multiple correlation coefficient between Y (i.e., the dependent variable, such as number of daily deaths) and the X's (i.e., pollution, weather and other independent variables) when these are correctly measured, and R_e^2, the corresponding value when errors of measurement are present. In general, three types of error structure can be possible. If the observed variable Z (say, ambient PM concentrations) is related to the true value of exposure X (say, personal PM exposures) according to:

$$Z = X + E \qquad (4\text{-}3)$$

where E is the assumed error (uncertainty) in the measurement of X. It is assigned a mean value of zero with a standard deviation. Three types of measurement error can be considered depending on the nature of correlation ("corr") between these three variables (Wacholder, 1995):

■ Classical Error if corr(X, E) = 0

■ Berkson Error of corr(Z, E) = 0

■ General Error Model if corr(X, E) ≠ 0

In regression analysis with only one independent variable the classical error in that variable will cause bias towards the "null" (or zero) in the observed regression coefficient b, estimated from the model: $Y = \alpha + bZ +$ error. The relation between b and the true regression coefficient B (i.e. from the model $Y = \alpha + BX +$ error) is given by: $b =$ BIAS $\times$ B, where BIAS (or the reliability coefficient according to Cochran [1970] and Lebret [1990]) is defined as:

$$\text{BIAS} = \frac{\text{Var}(X)}{\text{Var}(X) + \text{Var}(E)} = \frac{\sigma^2}{\sigma^2 + w^2} \qquad (4\text{-}4)$$

According to Lebret (1990) and also Wacholder (1995) in the "Berkson case," regression with one independent variable will not lead to a bias in estimating B or the exposure-response relationship. In both cases, however, the measurement errors or exposure uncertainties will reduce the statistical power of the analysis making it difficult to detect a true underlying association between exposures and health effects. When there are more exposure variables and other confounders in the regression model (such as weather, SES and other pollutants) the problem becomes more complicated. In addition to uncertainty in the surrogate exposure measure, correlation among the different exposure and weather variables will affect the degree of bias in the estimated regression coefficients. In this case, depending on the sign of the correlation between X and E the bias in the regression coefficient for the exposure variable may be toward or away from zero (Wacholder, 1995). Even though it is theoretically possible to overestimate the magnitude of the exposure-response relationship when exposure and confounding variables are correlated and/or a very poor exposure surrogate is used, such a finding is not typically expected. According to Wacholder (1995) this would require a strong negative correlation ($\rho < -0.5$) between error and true exposures and that the variance of the error be greater than the variance of the true value. Analysis of PTEAMS personal and outdoor 24-hour average PM concentrations showed that neither of these conditions were true. The bias calculated using average or daily outdoor PM_{10}, instead of the corresponding personal PM_{10} exposure values, was also not great (about 0.6). Furthermore, most time-series models of daily mortality or hospital admissions incorporate techniques of detrending the data either directly or indirectly (Özkaynak et al., 1993, Schwartz, 1996). In addition to removing most of the serial correlation in the data, these methods also reduce the correlation between the adjusted covariates. Hence, measurement error and cross-correlation problems are further reduced when variables are filtered or adjusted in the fitted regression models. In conclusion, measurement uncertainties and multicollinearity among the regression variables can influence the estimated PM_{10} health risk coefficients. In reality, however, these strong biases or "false positives" are not reasonably expected from either the cross-sectional or time-series epidemiologic models if they include sufficient adjustment for seasonality and key confounders.

Of course, the opposite problem of not being able to detect a hypothesized association is also likely when the study sample size is too small. For example, as stated in Xue et al. (1993), in ordinary or a logistic regression modeling setting, the study power is a function of both the sample size and the R^2 of the prediction model for the selected exposure variable (i.e., personal or indoor PM). In other words: $(Z_\beta + Z_{\alpha/2})^2$ is proportional to NR^2 (i.e. sample size times the regression coefficient of determination), where $Z_{\alpha/2}$ and Z_β (study power) are critical values of the normal distribution, with N being the sample size. Therefore, for a given study power N is proportional to $1/R^2$. Thus, when exposures are estimated, rather than directly measured, the sample size of an epidemiologic study has to be increased proportional to $1/R^2$ in order to maintain a desired level of power for being able to detect a hypothesized association. For example, if ambient PM values instead of the mean personal PM values were to be used in the statistical analysis of daily mortality data, the effective sample size needs to be increased by a factor of 3 or (1/0.32) if the relationship between mean personal PM and mean ambient PM is given as in Figure 4.4. In general, however, most time-series studies analyze multiple years of over 1000 daily records of mortality and morbidity data. In these instances, reduction of sample size becomes less of a problem if the R^2 for the personal exposure model on ambient PM measurements are not very small. For community average exposure-response analysis, an R^2 of around 0.3 for the personal exposure prediction model, as in the case of the PTEAM study, should be sufficient to detect a significant exposure-response coefficient based on few years of daily records. Consequently, an overwhelming majority of the epidemiologic studies to be summarized in Chapters 6 and 7 were able to estimate statistically significant PM_{10}—mortality coefficients based on analysis of two or more years of records of daily mortality.

Summary

Over the past fifteen years, much has been learned about the physical and chemical nature of airborne particulate matter, whether it is located indoors or outdoors. However, there is much less known about how these factors affect the potency of inhaled particles. We recognize that ambient PM contributes to indoor concentrations in conjunction with several factors such as air exchange rates and particle size. However, outdoor measurements at current levels are not strongly associated with personal exposures to particulate mass. Fine (respirable) particles and the components associated with them (e.g., acid aerosols, certain metals, and organic solvent extractable material) penetrate indoor spaces more readily than large particles. Under some conditions, measurements of respirable PM may represent a reasonable approximation of indoor and personal exposure to outdoor sources. Of course, indoor sources would not be represented by ambient measurements. Furthermore, fine particles and the acidic components they contain tend to be more homogeneously distributed throughout the outdoor environment in many communities, than TSP, PM_{10}, or coarse particles. The important components of personal exposures are received during contact with indoor sources, primarily found in homes and work places. Nevertheless, ambient aerosols still contribute about half or more of the personal PM exposures of most individuals in the general population. Because of the known toxicity of the many species of urban aerosols, the contribution of ambient aerosols to the total toxicity of inhaled particles is significant. Aside from environmental tobacco smoke and cooking generated aerosols, most indoor particles are not expected to be any more toxic than the outdoor particles. Of course, cat, cockroach, dog, mite, and other allergenic dust can evoke reactions in sensitized individuals. Therefore, based on size, mass and relative toxicity considerations, ambient particles are definitely an important concern in the investigation of health effects of exposures to respirable particles.

Despite decades of research and dozens of studies in support of the correlations between specific outdoor pollutant concentration levels and adverse health effects, there still remains an undercurrent of disbelief or concern as to the validity of the conclusions drawn from these studies. In particular, Lipfert and Wyzga (1995a) comment that the "availability and quality of observed data may limit the validity of the conclusions that can be derived...." Owing to the complex nature of ambient pollutant mixtures, this paper concludes that "differences in the reliability of exposure estimates can be critical in the implied relationships between correlated variables in multiple regressions." In addition, measurement error is alleged to obscure the true degree of co-linearity that may actually be present (Lipfert and Wyzga, 1995a). Clearly there is no question that better estimates of actual personal exposures are essential. However, as discussed above, use of ambient PM concentrations as a surrogate for personal exposures are not expected to change the essential results from past epidemiologic studies utilizing community average health and pollution data.

Lipfert and Wyzga (1995b) also question the fundamental process of multivariate statistical analysis. There is little recognition given to the level of scientific inquiry undertaken as many different types of statistical methods are applied to air pollution studies. Effectively, the authors discount any conclusions drawn whereby a single pollutant can be held "responsible" for specific health effects. Their analysis is committed to proving that hypothesis in spite of dozens of published studies that have collectively shown a positive and a statistically significant association with ambient particulates and daily mortality. Due to differences in the study locations, and hence the diversity in the composition of the pollution mix, it is nearly impossible for all of these studies to suffer from similar co-linearity problems, measurement uncertainties, and yet come up with a positive and statistically significant association. At this point we may not be very certain about the size of the effect, but we have little doubt that based on existing epidemiologic evidence that a significant and a positive particle effect on human health exists. This estimated effect persists even in models that simultaneously account for exposures to other pollutants in the atmosphere, such as CO, NO_2, O_3. The challenge that remains now is to identify the component or constituents of respirable particles that are responsible for the statistically detected health effects. Better instrumentation, better exposure monitoring, further speciation of indoor, outdoor, and personal aerosols, in conjunction with new cohort studies should be conducted in order to improve our current knowledge on particle health effects.

5

Animal Toxicology

Mary Amdur

Introduction

The results of toxicological studies on experimental animals provide one cornerstone of the data base needed to evaluate the health effects of air pollutants. The acute air pollution episodes in Donora and London in the late forties and early fifties provided needed impetus for research developments in this area. It was plain that the concentration gap between even the high levels of pollution occurring during those incidents and concentrations needed to produce a response in animals by the then conventional criteria of mortality and pulmonary pathology was too great to make such studies of practical value. Over the ensuing decades pulmonary toxicologists have responded to this challenge by developing criteria that are both sensitive and biologically relevant to responses observed in people exposed to pollution. It is possible to examine response in experimental animals at concentrations at or near those that actually occur in ambient air.

It is important to evaluate animal toxicology as a predictive discipline by examining past successes and past failures in predicting human health effects. This chapter will address one of toxicology's outstanding success stories relating to the sulfur oxide–sulfuric acid pollution complex. Some of the data are very old, some are very new, but over the years the pieces of the jigsaw puzzle have gradually fitted together. The picture that emerges is one of amazing consistency that points clearly to sulfuric acid as the pollutant of main concern. Across the board, the animal and human data are mutually supportive.

To put the toxicological studies in perspective, it is necessary to examine some of the peak concentrations of sulfuric acid that have been reported. If toxicological studies require levels vastly in excess of these concentrations to produce detectable effects, data so obtained have minimal predictive value. Measurements made in a smelter area in 1950–51 indicated that the concentration of sulfuric acid never exceeded 400 µg/m³ with an average value of 20 µg/m³ and in 1950, concentrations up to 240 µg/m³ were found in the Los Angeles area (Amdur et al. 1952). In a ten-year study in London from 1954–1964, the highest daily average was 347 µg/m³ and the highest hourly average was 678 µg/m³ during an episode in December 1962 (Commins and Waller 1967). In 1963 daily measurements were started in London. The 24-hour values are shown in Table 5.1 for the winter months of Nov.–Feb. (Ito and Thurston 1989). These levels are comparable to, or above, typical levels in animal studies.

For reasons that are frankly incomprehensible to this author, measurements of sulfuric acid almost ceased everywhere for a decade or more. This was indeed unfortunate and, as toxicology indicated, made the results of sophisticated epidemiology studies much less definitive than they otherwise would have been. Fortunately, measurements of sulfuric acid are now being made. Peak values in excess of 20–40 µg/m³ lasting from 1 to 12 hours have been observed (Lioy and Waldman 1989). During a study done in Ontario in the summer of 1986, an hour-long peak of 50 µg/m³ was observed (Spengler et al. 1989). These values are much lower than the historic values discussed above. As we shall see,

TABLE 5.1

Historical London Daily Aerosol Acidity Data, Winter Months (Nov.–Feb.), 24-hour Average

Year	Sulfuric Acid µg/m³	
	Avg.	Max.
1963/64	10.4	134.1
1964/65	7.3	42.2
1965/66	7.5	24.3
1966/67	5.2	22.5
1967/68	7.6	25.3
1968/69	6.0	17.0
1969/70	4.8	19.0
1970/71	3.3	29.7
1971/72	4.5	13.7

Data from Ito and Thurston (1979).

however, a variety of toxicological studies show effects at concentrations of this order of magnitude.

Comparative Toxicity of Sulfur Dioxide and Sulfuric Acid

Down through the years, the main focus of epidemiological research on the sulfur compounds was sulfur dioxide. In the early days, this was quite understandable but it continued beyond its time. Fortunately, at long last, that emphasis in epidemiological studies has shifted to sulfuric acid as toxicology had been indicating for nearly two decades should be done. Table 5.2 examines the comparative irritant potency of sulfur dioxide and sulfuric acid that was determined by various criteria in two species of animals and in human subjects. To make the comparison, concentrations of sulfur dioxide and sulfuric acid have been expressed as $\mu mols/m^3$ of the two compounds. A study of Table 5.2 indicates that these pieces of the jigsaw puzzle fit together very well. The animal data obtained by measurement of airway resistance in guinea pigs and of bronchial clearance of particles in donkeys predicted that sulfuric acid was more irritant by at least an order of magnitude than sulfur dioxide. The response of human subjects measured by altered bronchial clearance, decreased tidal volume and increased airway resistance confirmed this prediction. The greater irritant potency of sulfuric acid as compared to sulfur dioxide relates to the different manner of deposition, with high local concentrations occurring when the aerosol particle is deposited on the surface. The very major difference noted in the bronchial clearance studies would also relate to the fact that the high concentrations of sulfur dioxide (300 ppm in donkeys and 13 ppm in human subjects) would be

TABLE 5.2

Comparative Acute Toxicity of SO_2 and H_2SO_4 ($\mu mol/m^3$)

	SO_2	H_2SO_4	Reference
Guinea Pig—1 hr. 10% Incr. Airway Resistance	6	1	Amdur (1974)
Donkeys—30 min.–1hr. Altered Bronchial Clearance	8,875	2	Spiegelman et al. (1968) Schlesinger et al. (1978)
Normal subjects—1 hr. Altered Bronchial Clearance	520	1	Lippmann et al. (1976) Leikauf et al. (1981)
Normal Subjects—10 min. 5% Decreased Tidal Volume	29	1	Amdur (1954)
Adolescent Asthmatics—40 min. Equal Incr. Airway Resistance	20	1	Koenig et al. (1989)

removed by the upper respiratory tract whereas the 0.3 μm sulfuric acid particle would penetrate to the critical area.

The comparative data discussed above were all obtained from acute exposures of an hour or less. The next question to ask is whether these acute studies are predictive of the comparative response to chronic long term exposures. Table 5.3 shows the results of two year studies on monkeys exposed to 1 ppm (41 μmols /m^3) sulfur dioxide or to 480 μg/m^3 (5 μmols/m^3) sulfuric acid. Once again, the data are given as μmols/m^3 of the two compounds for comparison. In the chronic studies, as in the acute studies, sulfuric acid was the more potent irritant. Obviously such chronic exposures cannot be done on human subjects but it is reasonable to assume, based on the similarity of animals and man in the acute studies which correctly predicted the relative potency in chronic studies, that sulfuric acid would be the more potent substance in man as well as in the monkeys. Current findings in epidemiological studies certainly support this assumption.

Response of Guinea Pigs with High Airway Resistance

When levels of air pollutants rise, the individuals most seriously affected are those with pre-existing cardiopulmonary disease. This has been shown for current levels of pollution by studies of hospital admissions of such patients (Bates and Sizto 1989). General admissions did not rise, but admissions related to respiratory disease did. That asthmatics are particularly sensitive was suggested by the fact that 88 percent of asthmatics had exacerbation of their symptoms during the Donora incident (Schrenk et al. 1949). Does animal toxicology have anything to offer that fits with these observations? The answer is yes it does in the form of a spin-off from my long term use of increase in airway resistance in guinea pigs as a standard bioassay to evaluate the response to irritants (Amdur 1964).

In the experimental design used, control measurements on each animal were made followed by measurements during a one-hour exposure to

TABLE 5.3

Comparative Chronic Toxicity of SO$_2$ and H$_2$SO$_4$, Monkeys—Two Years (μmol/m^3)

	SO$_2$	H$_2$SO$_4$	Reference
No Effect	41	None	Alarie et al. (1972)
Histopathology, Lowered Arterial O$_2$; Distribution of Ventilation	None	5	Alarie et al. (1975)

the irritant. Control and exposure data were thus available on about a thousand animals. Some of them had been exposed to irritant gases or vapors alone, some to combinations of irritant gas and inert aerosol and some to irritant aerosol. These data were examined to see if animals that had control (pre-exposure) airway resistance values in the upper range showed a greater change in response to irritants than did the remainder of the animals. If this was the case, it was then of further interest to see how concentration and type of irritant exposure impacted upon the response.

These animals were divided into 102 groups on the basis of the exposure received. As a starting point the groups were examined for animals showing a control resistance of 0.90 cm H_2O/ml/sec or greater. The choice of this value as the dividing line was based quite simply on the fact that, from long experience, my assistants and I regarded such a value as "high," yet we saw it often enough that a sample of sufficient size for statistical treatment would probably be obtained. When the data were finally analyzed this value was found to be more than one standard deviation removed from the group mean.

The control data are shown in Table 5.4. Of the 102 exposure groups, 68 contained at least one animal with a high resistance. These 68 tables included 734 animals. Table 5.5 shows a further examination of these 68 groups. They contained 135 animals with high resistance values with an average control resistance of 0.98 cm H_2O/ml/sec. Thus about 13% of the total population of 1,028 animals fell into this sub-group.

Table 5.6 shows the effect of high control (pre-exposure) resistance on the degree of response to an irritant expressed as the ratio of the resistance increase observed in the high resistance animals compared with that for the remainder of the group. For all the irritants taken together, the first row shows that there is a greater response if the control resistance was high. The second row shows that when the irritant was a gas or vapor there was no difference in response between the two sub-groups. On the other hand, when an irritant aerosol (either sulfuric acid or zinc ammo-

TABLE   5.4

Control Resistance (R) (Pre-Exposure Resistance)

	No High R	With High R	Total
Exposure Groups	34	68	102
Number of Animals	294	734	1028
Average Resistance (cm H_2O/(ml/sec))	0.68	0.76	0.73

TABLE 5.5
Control Resistance of 68 Groups Containing at Least One High Resistance Animal

	Normal R	High R	Total
Number of Animals	599	135	734
Average Resistance (cm H_2O/ml/sec)	0.70	0.98	0.76

TABLE 5.6
Effect of High Control (Pre-Exposure) Resistance on Response

	No. of Animals		Response Ratio
Exposure	High R	Normal R	High/Normal
All Irritants	135	599	1.44[a]
Irritant Gas	41	204	1.04
Irritant Aerosol	18	85	1.73[c]
Gas + Aerosol	76	310	1.63[b]
Major Response	47	141	1.28
Slight Response	37	187	1.85[c]
Ten highest	10	82	2.09[b]

[a] $p < 0.001$
[b] $p < 0.01$
[c] $p < 0.05$

nium sulfate) was present or when an inert aerosol was present with an irritant gas, thus forming an irritant aerosol, the response was greater in the high resistance group. This is really an important point and fits with the fact that aerosols can be more potent irritants than gases as was indicated earlier by the comparative irritant potency of sulfuric acid and sulfur dioxide. Delivery as an aerosol produces high local concentrations. The response to an irritant gas sorbed on an inert aerosol is less rapidly reversible than the response to the irritant gas alone.

The next factor examined was whether the animals with high pre-exposure resistance would show a greater response to irritant exposures of sufficient magnitude to more than double the airway resistance in the average group. There was no difference between the response of the high resistance and the normal animals in those groups. This suggests that concentrations sufficient to produce such changes overwhelm any effects of the pre-exposure high control resistance. This too may be an important point in that it reinforces the fact that *extrapolation from higher doses is basically not appropriate to air pollution toxicology.* When the response produced had been slight, the response of the animals with high pre-exposure (control) resistance was 1.85 times the normal response (row 6 of Table 5.6). At low concentrations this added stress becomes of importance and this concept fits well with the related observations of hospital admissions of persons with respiratory impairment. The next question asked was how did the response of the ten animals with the highest control resistance (an average of 1.23 with a range of 1.12 to 1.40 cm $H_2O/(ml/sec)$) compare with the average response? Their response was twice that of the average.

If we accept the fact that the high resistance guinea pigs are more sensitive to low level exposures and the fact that the most sensitive animals are the ten with the highest resistance, it then becomes of interest to see if any of these ten fall into the low level exposure category. Three of them did and the data are shown in Table 5.7. The response ranged from 4 to nearly 10 times the normal response of the animals in this exposure sub-group (smaller group then the animals in Table 5.5). These animals under these conditions of minimal exposure appear to be the analog of the sensitive individuals who react to acute air pollution incidents.

The Response of Asthmatics to Sulfur Pollution

Back in 1970, it was suggested that the Amdur-Mead guinea pig model was analogous to the response of the sensitive segment of the population (Amdur 1970). In the 1980s data on the response of exercising asthmatics to extremely low levels of sulfur dioxide began to appear from the University of California at San Francisco and the University of Washington. The reporting of these data livened up the meetings of the Environmental Protection Agency's Clean Air Scientific Advisory Committee no end; the desperate efforts to shoot down the data were believ-

TABLE 5.7

Response to Levels of Irritant—Animals with Highest Control (Pre-Exposure Resistance)

Control Resistance Cm H$_2$O/(ml/sec)		Change Cm H$_2$O/(ml/sec)		Response Ratio
High	Normal	High	Normal	High/Normal
1.29	0.69	2.04	0.51	4.00
1.15	0.74	1.40	0.24	6.36
1.13	0.74	2.16	0.22	9.80

able only to an experienced and hardened cynic. It was not surprising when additional data simply strengthened the initial findings. As shown in Table 5.8, the guinea pig data had predicted it quantitatively. These findings on asthmatic subjects have an important impact and require that we rethink the importance of short-term peak levels of sulfur dioxide. In the 1970s, we were ready to dismiss it as a pollutant which *per se* could not cause adverse health effects at concentrations that occur in the atmosphere. That *cannot now be done*, a point well made by Sheppard (1988).

Data are now available on the response of asthmatics to sulfuric acid (Utell et al. 1984; Koenig et al. 1989). As with sulfur dioxide, asthmatics, especially adolescent asthmatics are more sensitive than normal subjects. Table 5.9 indicates that once again the Amdur-Mead guinea pig model had predicted such a response (Amdur et al. 1978). Koenig et al. (1989) reported that although 0.1 ppm (260 $\mu g/m^3$) sulfur dioxide did not produce a response, it did increase the response to 68 $\mu g/m^3$ sulfuric acid when the gas at 0.1 ppm was given with the sulfuric acid aerosol. This is an important observation because both pollutants can occur together and impact on a sensitive segment of the population.

TABLE   5 . 8

From Guinea Pig to Man—Sulfur Dioxide

Guinea Pigs	0.2–1 ppm cause slight but statistically significant readily reversible increase in airway resistance
Normal Human Subjects	5 ppm is needed to produce statistically significant increase in airway resistance
Exercising Asthmatics	0.25–1 ppm cause slight but statistically significant readily reversible increase in airway resistance

TABLE   5 . 9

From Guinea Pig to Man—Sulfuric Acid

Guinea Pigs	100–1000 $\mu g/m^3$ for 1 hour causes dose-related increase in airway resistance (Amdur 1978)
Normal Human Subjects	1000 $\mu g/m^3$ causes no response (Many studies)
Adult Exercising Asthmatics	450–1000 $\mu g/m^3$ for 16 min. causes dose-related increase in airway resistance; 100 $\mu g/m^3$ causes no response (Utell et al. 1984)
Adolescent Exercising Asthmatics	68–100 $\mu g/m^3$ for 40 min with 10 min exercise causes increase in airway resistance (Koenig 1989)

Effects of Sulfuric Acid on Bronchial Mucociliary Clearance

Another important action of sulfuric acid is an alteration in the mucociliary clearance of particles from the bronchial area of the lung. Data are available on donkeys and rabbits as well as on human subjects. The animal data have been highly predictive of the response observed in the human subjects.

Table 5.10 shows the effects of sulfuric acid on mucociliary clearance in donkeys and human subjects. In short exposures clearance was slowed in donkeys and also in human subjects by a concentration of 1000 µg/m³. At a concentration of 100 µg/m³ the clearance in human subjects was accelerated rather than decreased. In chronic exposures of donkeys for 6 months to 100 µg/m³ given 1 hr/day, 5 days/wk highly variable clearance rates and a persistent shift from base line clearance values were observed during exposure and for three months following the last exposure (Schlesinger et al. 1979). The effects of single short-term exposures to sulfuric acid on mucociliary clearance are similar in the two species. In donkeys, repeated exposure to low levels of sulfuric acid has a profound effect on clearance rates. It is neither ethical nor practical to do such repeated exposures in human subjects. It is, however, reasonable to assume that the chronic effects in human subjects would resemble those seen in the donkey.

TABLE 5.10

Mucociliary Clearance—Donkey and Man

	Sulfuric Acid Exposure (µg/m³)	Direction of Change
Donkeys—1 hr	200–1000	Decrease
Man	100	Increase
	1000	Decrease
Donkeys—6 mo 1 hr/day, 5 day/wk	100	Highly variable; Persisted 3 mo. post-exposure
	Cigarette Smoke	
Donkeys	2 Cigarettes	Increase
	15 Cigarettes	Decrease
Man	2 Cigarettes	Increase
Donkeys	30 Cigarettes 3 x/wk, 6 mo.	DECREASE
Man	Heavy Smokers	DECREASE

Capitalized DECREASE indicates a considerable change.

This assumption is further strengthened by the data for exposure to cigarette smoke also shown in Table 5.10. The acute response to cigarette smoke is strikingly similar in donkeys and human subjects (Lippman et al. 1982). Furthermore, the chronic exposure of donkeys to cigarette smoke resulted in a profound slowing of clearance. This same response is seen in heavy smokers, whose clearance rate is greatly reduced. The similarity of the chronic response of the donkeys to both irritants suggests that this would be true also of human subjects.

Figure 5.1 shows the effects on bronchial mucociliary clearance in rabbits and human subjects exposed for 1 hour to graded concentrations of sulfuric acid (Shlesinger et al. 1984). In the rabbit, 100 µg/m³ had no effect, 200–300 µg/m³ accelerated clearance, and 1000–2000 µg/m³ produced a slowing of clearance. The human subjects were more sensitive than the rabbits since a concentration of 100 µg/m³ accelerated clearance. The same concentration dependence of effect seen in the rabbits was observed in the human subjects as 1000 µg/m³ produced a slowing in clearance.

Effects on Rabbits of Chronic Exposure to Sulfuric Acid

Data are available on chronic exposure of rabbits 1 hr/day, 5 days/week for periods of 4, 8 and 12 months to 250 µg/m³ sulfuric acid (Gearhart and Shlesinger 1989). One group of animals was examined after a 3 month recovery period following the 12 month exposure. Some of the results of these studies are shown in Table 5.11. A variety of criteria in

T A B L E   5 . 1 1

Effects of Chronic Exposure of Rabbits to Sulfuric Acid, 250 µg/m³, 1 hr/day, 5 day/wk

End Point	Exposure			Post-Exposure
	4 mo	8 mo	12 mo	3 mo
Mucociliary Clearance	Decrease	Decrease	Decrease	DECREASE
Airway Sensitivity	Increase	INCREASE	INCREASE	nm
Airway Diameter	Decrease	Decrease	DECREASE	mc
Secretory Cell Number	Increase	INCREASE	INCREASE	INCREASE
Secretory Cell pH	Decrease	Decrease	Decrease	Decrease

Capitalized INCREASE and DECREASE means a considerable change.
nm: not measured
nc: no change
Data from Gearhart and Schlesinger (1989).

FIGURE 5.1

Exposure-Dependent Changes in Bronchial Mucociliary Clearance Times in Rabbits (Mean Residence Time) and Humans (Clearance Halftime) Due to 1 Hour Exposure to Submicrometer H₂SO₄ Aerosols

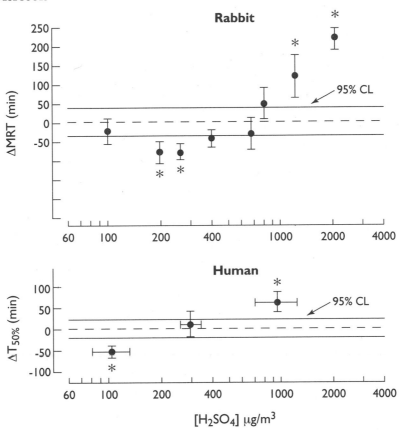

Vertical bars are ±S.E. for group mean. Horizontal bands are mean ±1 S.E. of measurements of sham controls. Asterisks indicate significant change (p<0.05).

Data from Schlesinger, Chen and Driscoll, 1984.

addition to bronchial mucociliary clearance were used to evaluate response. These criteria were carefully chosen to be relevant to human disease. Slowing of bronchial mucociliary clearance occurred during the first week of exposure, became progressive after the 19th week of exposure and was still present 3 months after the exposure had been terminated. This delayed recovery is consistent with earlier data cited above on donkeys.

The airways became progressively sensitive to challenge with acetylcholine indicating that sulfuric acid had increased bronchial reactivity. There was a progressive decrease in airway diameter accompanied by an increase in the number of secretory cells, especially in the smaller airways. Acidic glycoprotein content of mucus increased. The lowered pH of secretory cells and mucus is especially important. The implications of this have been reviewed by Holma (1989). The changes observed in these studies are of importance because similar changes have been associated with both chronic bronchitis and asthma. When one considers the similarity of the 1-hour response of rabbits and human subjects, it is reasonable to regard these data as predictive of the response that would be observed in human subjects were such a protocol possible. The potential implications of these findings for the role of sulfuric acid as a contributor to the development of chronic bronchitis in exposed populations are discussed by Lippmann et al. (1987).

Sulfuric Acid Sorbed on Metal Oxide Particles

If toxicology is to be usefully predictive, it must examine not only low concentrations but also specific types of particles known to occur. The jigsaw puzzle of the sulfuric acid story is an interdisciplinary problem and unless particle-complex is thoroughly understood there is little hope of eventually putting it together.

Field studies as well as laboratory research have shown that some of the sulfuric acid in the atmosphere is sorbed on ultrafine metal oxide particles emitted by smelting operations and combustion of coal. As much as 9% of the sulfur present in certain coals may be emitted from the stack in this form (Amdur et al. 1986). There are also indications that the metals catalyzing the conversion of sulfur dioxide to sulfuric acid are concentrated in the ultrafine (< 0.1 µm) particles (Davidson et al. 1974). Furthermore these metals tend to be concentrated on the surface of particles (Linton et al. 1976) This has been observed in both field and laboratory studies. The toxicological significance of these facts is that even though these concentrations of sulfuric acid may be very low they would reach the deep lung carried on the surface of ultrafine particles and thus be available to produce significant physiological, biochemical and morphological damage in a critical area of the lung. The lack of toxicological information on such particles was a major gap in the sulfur oxide–particulate matter data base. A ten year program at Massachusetts Institute of Technology involving toxicologists, pathologists, metallurgists and combustion engineers working together at the bench level provided data on the response to these particles as well as fundamental information on the mechanisms of their formation.

In order to examine the response to such particles it is evident that freshly generated particles must be used. Collected and resuspended fly ash would for a number of reasons be *completely useless*. Resuspension of the ultrafine mode poses very difficult problems and, more importantly, the layer of sulfuric acid would not survive collection, storage and resuspension. High temperature furnaces that could be adapted as feed systems for animal exposure chambers were used to produce either ultrafine metal oxides or coal combustion aerosols under carefully controlled conditions.

The prototype aerosol used in these studies was 0.05 μm zinc oxide with sorbed sulfuric acid. Details of the generation and characterization of the aerosol and the pulmonary response have been reported in detail (Amdur et al. 1986, 1988,1989, McCarthy et al. 1982). The guinea pig was the experimental animal. The toxicological criteria used were chosen to examine mainly effects in the alveolar regions of the lung where such particles are deposited. One of the most useful of these is measurement of diffusing capacity of carbon monoxide (DL_{CO}). A decrease in DL_{CO} indicates an impairment of oxygenation of the blood across the alveolar-capillary membrane.

Concentrations of zinc oxide of 1, 2.5 or 5 mg/m^3 were used to deliver sorbed concentrations of sulfuric acid of 20, 30 or 60 μg/m^3. A single 3-hour exposure to these aerosols caused a dose-related decrease in DL_{CO} that correlated with the amount of sulfuric acid sorbed on the particles. At 20 μg/m^3 sulfuric acid there was no effect. At concentrations of 30 μg/m^3 or greater there was a statistically significant reduction in DL_{CO}. A concentration of 60 μg/m^3 caused a reduction of DL_{CO} of about 50% and at 72 hours after this single 3-hour exposure, DL_{CO} was still 15–20% below control values. As shown in Figure 5.2, this persistent decrease in DL_{CO} was accompanied by other slowly reversible changes in compartments of lung volume and increased levels of cells, protein and a variety of enzymes in lavage fluid.

Increased levels of angiotensin converting enzyme in the plasma provide an indication of damage to endothelial cells. A single exposure to 30 or to 160 μg/m^3 sorbed sulfuric acid produced respectively 20% and 58% increases above control values. Damage to airway epithelial cells may be shown by increased permeability to intratracheally injected horseradish peroxidase, The above exposures produced respectively increases of 62 and 146% above control. These findings indicate that the degree of damage to endothelial and epithelial cells is also dose related.

FIGURE 5.2

Effects on Guinea Pigs (8 per Group) of Single 3-Hour Exposure to 60 µg/m³ H₂SO₄ Sorbed on Ultrafine ZnO Aerosol As Evaluated by Pulmonary Function and Enzymes, Cells and Protein in Lung Lavage Fluid

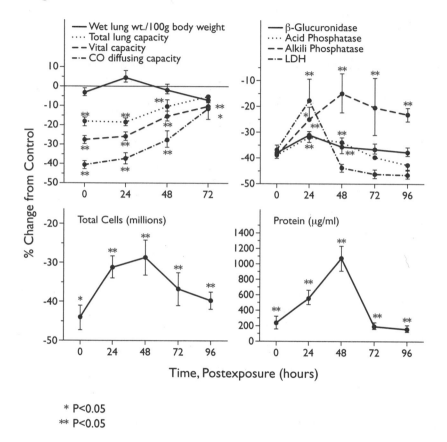

Time, Postexposure (hours)

* P<0.05
** P<0.05

Data from Amdur and Chen, 1989.

Evidence of morphological damage in the centriacinar region of the lung paralleled these functional and biological changes. The overall pattern of changes was very similar to results obtained with ozone, another deep lung irritant (Miller et al. 1987). In the lungs of guinea pigs exposed for 3 hours to 50 µg/m³ sorbed sulfuric acid there was distention of the perivascular and peribronchial connective tissues which was interpreted as pulmonary edema. This was confirmed by electron microscopy and an increase in lung weight. The alveolar interstitium also appeared distended.

The changes were seen in 83% of animals studied immediately or 12 hours after exposure but had reversed by 48 hours after exposure.

As indicated above, a single 3-hour exposure to 20 µg/m³ did not affect pulmonary function and the effects of 30 µg/m³ were slight. The results of repeated exposures of 3 hr/day for 5 days to these two concentrations are shown in Figure 5.3. Compartments of lung volume and

---

FIGURE 5.3

Effect of Repeated Daily 3-Hour Exposures on Total Lung Capacity, Vital Capacity, Diffusing Capacity, and Wet Lung Weight to Body Weight Ratios, Measured Immediately After Exposure

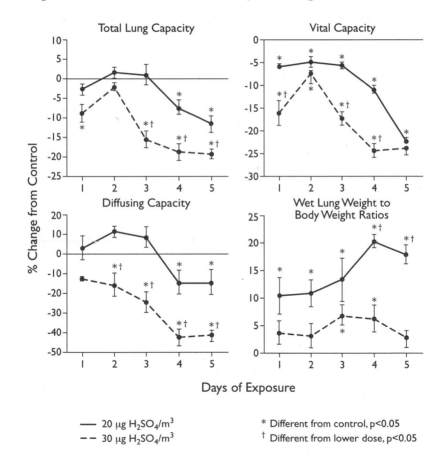

Days of Exposure

— 20 µg H₂SO₄/m³

-- 30 µg H₂SO₄/m³

* Different from control, p<0.05

† Different from lower dose, p<0.05

Values are mean ± SE for eight guinea pigs.
Data from Amdur and Chen, 1989.

DL_{CO} decreased as exposure continued and lung weight-body weight ratio increased. These effects were both progressive and dose related. The relationship between the decrease in DL_{CO} and the cumulative dose of sorbed sulfuric acid was examined. The cumulative dose was obtained by multiplying the measured concentration of sulfur with valence (S^{VI}) for each 3 hours by three and summing them. The results shown in Figure 5.4 indicate that the observed response was related to the cumulative dose.

Animals that had been exposed to 20 μg/m³ of sulfuric acid 3 hr/day for 5 days were rested on days 6 and 7. When pulmonary function was measured on day 8 the values had returned to control. Animals were then again exposed for 3 hours on days 8 and 9. No change was seen on day 8 but on day 9 the values fell abruptly to levels observed at the end of the 5 day exposure. Table 5.12 shows the data obtained for DL_{CO} and total

F I G U R E   5 . 4

Reduction in CO Diffusing Capacity Plotted Against Cumulative Dose of S^{VI}

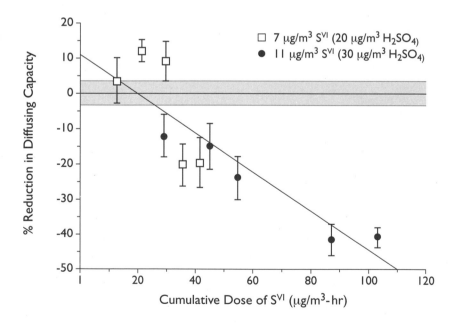

Shaded area indicates 95% confidence limits.
Data from Amdur, Chen and Guty, 1988.

TABLE 5.12

Increased Lung Sensitivity from 5-Day Exposure to Sorbed Sulfuric Acid, 20 µg/m³, 3 hr/day

Day	% Change from Control	
	DL$_{CO}$	TLC
1–3	N.C.	N.C.
5	-15%	-12%
6–7	Rest: No Exposure or Measurements	
8	N.C.	N.C.
9	-18%	-15%

N.C. = No Change

lung capacity (TLC). Even though the parameters of respiratory function were completely normal following the two day rest, the lung had become more sensitive to reexposure.

In addition to the sulfuric acid sorbed on ultrafine zinc oxide, studies were made on the response to the ultrafine fraction of ash produced by carefully controlled coal combustion. Analytical chemistry studies have shown that the ultrafine ash from combustion of Illinois No. 6 coal carried sorbed sulfuric acid and that the ash from Montana Lignite, a more alkaline coal, carried sorbed neutralized sulfate. The hypothesis was that the acidic ash from Illinois No. 6 would be much more irritant than the neutral ash from Montana Lignite. Figure 5.5 shows the data obtained in 2-hour exposures to these two coals (Chen et al. 1990). Even though the total sulfate was much higher in the Montana Lignite ash, the acidic Illinois No. 6 ash was much more irritant.

The fly ash produced in these laboratory studies resembles the primary emission from a coal burning power plant. Exposure to this emission could produce adverse health effects. For example in the Chestnut Ridge region of Pennsylvania an increased prevalence of wheeze in nonsmokers was observed in a population living downwind from a coal burning plant (Shenker et al. 1983). Although sulfuric acid was not measured in this study, the increase of wheeze was independently associated with increased sulfur dioxide concentration. Elevated sulfur dioxide levels downwind would be expected to be a surrogate indicator of sulfuric acid in the plume effluent. Once again the animal data appear to have relevance to observed health effects.

FIGURE 5.5

Response of 8 Guinea Pigs to 2-Hour Exposures

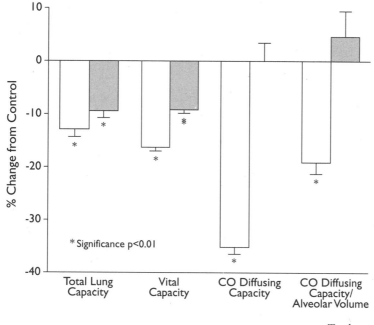

Coal Type	mg/m³	ppm SO₂	Total Sulfate µg/m³
☐ Illinois No. 6	6.33	1.36[†]	216
▨ Montana Liginite	8.67	0.3	2039

[†] SO₂ denuded

Data from Chen et al. 1990.

Comparison of Free and Sorbed Sulfuric Acid

It is possible to compare the response produced by sulfuric acid of equivalent particle size as a free mist or sorbed on either the zinc oxide particles or on the ultrafine Illinois No. 6 fly ash. Such comparative data are shown in Table 5.13 using the amount needed to reduce DL_{CO} 25% below control in exposures of 2 or 3 hours. Approximately ten times as much free acid of the same particle size was required to produce the response compared to the acid present sorbed on either zinc oxide or ultrafine coal fly ash. The fourth column expresses the results in terms of dose, as $(µg/m^3) \times hr$, needed to reduce DL_{CO} 25% below control. The final column is the slope of a line relating DL_{CO} with dose. The values for the two types of particles with sorbed sulfuric acid are very close.

TABLE 5.13

Relative Potency of Free and Sorbed Sulfuric Acid, in Reducing DL_{CO} 25% Below Control

Exposure	C $\mu g/m^3$	Time (T) (hours)	Total (C × T) $(\mu g/m^3) \times hr$	Slope $[(\mu g/m^3) \times hr]^{-1}$
Free Acid	310	3	930	0.03
ZnO Sorbed	30	3	90	0.28
Illinois No. 6 coal	43	2	86	0.29

In longer exposures of 3 hr/day, 5 days/wk for 4 weeks Illinois No. 6 and fine (0.3 μm) free sulfuric acid showed minimal effects on pulmonary function. Slight effects were seen with ultrafine (0.03 μm) free sulfuric. In terms of percent change from control per $\mu eq/m^3$ of H^+ the sulfuric acid sorbed on zinc oxide was ten times as irritant as the ultrafine sulfuric acid. This greater irritant potency of the sulfuric acid sorbed on zinc oxide is in agreement with the earlier data from short term single exposures.

Joint Action of Sulfuric Acid and Ozone

The question of the potential for joint toxic action of ozone and sulfuric acid is one of considerable importance. Both pollutants are present in the summer air pollution that occurs in the Northeast as well as in other air pollution situations. Studies of hospital admissions for respiratory related disorders and studies of pulmonary function in children attending summer camps join to suggest that the concentration of both pollutants is an important determinant of the observed response. The data available on the response of animals to these pollutants either combined or given in sequential exposures indicate that the results can depend upon the mode and duration of exposure and perhaps upon the nature of the sulfuric acid (i.e. free or sorbed as well as on particle size) and upon the end point chosen as an assessment of response. In some studies the result has been an increase of the response expected from ozone alone; in others the result has been an attenuation of a response produced by one of the compounds given alone.

The response of guinea pigs to sulfuric acid sorbed on zinc oxide bears a striking resemblance to responses produced by ozone (Miller et al. 1987). These factors include decreases in compartments of lung volume and DL_{CO}, increased bronchial sensitivity and epithelial permeability to horseradish peroxidase, and morphological lesions in the centriacinar region of the lung. This led us to wonder if these aerosols would alter the response to subsequent exposures to ozone (Chen et al. 1991). A concentration of 0.15 ppm ozone was chosen for these experiments because earlier work had shown that it did not affect compartments of lung volume or DL_{CO}. Animals were exposed to furnace gases, 24 or 84 µg/m³ sorbed sulfuric acid for 1 hour. Two hours later they were exposed for 1 hour to either air or 0.15 ppm ozone. Vital capacity was reduced by the ozone following pre-exposure to 24 µg/m³ but DL_{CO} was not. Pre-exposure to the higher concentration resulted in decreases in both VC and DL_{CO} by the ozone exposure.

As was indicated earlier, a 3 hr/day 5 day exposure to 20 µg/m³ followed by a two day rest rendered the apparently normal lung more sensitive to subsequent exposure to the same concentration of sorbed acid. A similar experiment in which the guinea pigs were exposed 3 hr/day for 5 days to either furnace gases or 24 µg/m³ sorbed sulfuric acid, rested on days 6–8 and exposed on day 9 to 0.15 ppm ozone for an hour indicated that the lung was now more sensitive to ozone. In the animals pre-exposed to sorbed sulfuric acid but not in control animals pre-exposed to furnace gases alone, VC and DL_{CO} were reduced by the ozone exposure. Another piece of evidence that sulfuric acid can increase the sensitivity of the lung comes from the work of Osebold et al. (1980). They reported that ozone enhanced the allergic sensitivity of mice to inhaled antigen and that this action was potentiated by the presence of sulfuric acid.

With sensitive biochemical criteria of lung damage such as increased lung protein content or apparent increased collagen synthesis Last's group has accumulated evidence that quite low levels of sulfuric acid will potentiate the response to low levels of ozone in the rat (Last et al. 1984, 1989). In a 5 day exposure, the response to 0.2 ppm ozone was increased by 40 µg/m³. In 9 day exposures 20 µg/m³ produced a significant potentiation of the response to 0.2 ppm ozone. At 5 µg/m³, only a trend towards potentiation was seen suggesting that this is at or near the threshold level. The pollutant levels used in these studies are at or near to levels known to occur in the atmosphere. It should be noted that ammonium sulfate was also capable of potentiating the response to ozone but much higher concentrations were required: 5 mg/m³ potentiated the response, but 1 mg/m³ did not. It should also be emphasized that the interaction between ozone and these aerosols is clearly one in which the damaging effects of ozone on the centriacinar region of the lung are enhanced. The acid aerosols potentiate the effects of ozone and not *vice versa*. One hypothesis suggested to explain this effect involves increased lifetimes of free radicals at the sites of ozone interaction with the deep lung in more acidic environments.

The effect of particle size of the sulfuric acid on the joint response to ozone and sulfuric acid has been examined by Kimmel et al. (1994). Rats were exposed 4 hr/day for 2 days to filtered air, 500 µg/m^3 sulfuric acid of 0.3 or 0.06 µm, 0.6 ppm ozone and to the combination of ozone and acid. Twenty hours after the last exposure, the lungs were fixed and the lesion density, defined as the volume fraction of total parenchyma that contained markedly thickened alveolar septae, was measured by light microscopy. The ozone produced an increased lesion density but neither acid exposure alone produced a change from control. The ultrafine acid combined with ozone produced an increase greater than that seen with ozone alone but the fine acid did not alter the ozone response. Particle size of the acid may thus be a determinant in the effect of sulfuric acid on the response to ozone.

The synergistic action of sulfuric acid on the ozone response observed in the rat is interesting because the rat is one of the least sensitive species to effects of sulfuric acid. In the experiments of Last and his colleagues discussed earlier and those of the Kimmel et al. study the sulfuric acid alone produced no response. The guinea pig and the rabbit, on the other hand, show changes from exposure to either agent alone.

Rabbits received 3-hour exposures to sulfuric acid at 50, 75 or 125 µg/m^3 and 0.1, 0.3 or 0.6 ppm ozone alone or in combination (Schlesinger et al. 1992a). Following exposure bronchopulmonary lavage was performed. The pulmonary response endpoints chosen related to general cytotoxicity and macrophage function. Phagocytic activity of macrophages was depressed at the two highest acid concentrations and at all concentrations of ozone. Exposure to all mixtures showed significant antagonism. Superoxide production by stimulated macrophages was depressed by acid exposure at the two highest concentrations but ozone alone had no effect. Significant antagonism was observed when 0.1 or 0.3 ppm ozone was added to these acid levels. The activity of tumor necrosis factor elicited from stimulated macrophages was depressed by the two higher acid levels, but was unaffected by ozone. In this case, exposures to mixtures of 125 µg/m^3 with 0.3 or 0.6 ppm ozone resulted in a synergistic interaction. This study showed that whether the interaction between ozone and sulfuric acid was synergistic or antagonistic depended upon the end point chosen but the magnitude of the interaction was not always related to the concentrations of the constituent pollutants.

The effect of sulfuric acid on non-specific airway hyperresponsiveness was examined in rabbits exposed 3 hours to 50–500 µg/m^3 acid alone (El-Fawal et al. 1994), to 0.1–0.6 ppm ozone alone and to the combination of the two (Schlesinger et al. 1993). The assessment of response was made *in vitro* by administering increasing doses of acetylcholine to bronchial and tracheal rings obtained from exposed animals. In exposures to acid alone, bronchial reactivity was increased by acid concentrations of 75 $\mu g/m^3$ and above. The highest level, 500 $\mu g/m^3$, increased tracheal reactivity. This difference likely reflects the dosimetry as the 0.3 μm particles used would be mainly deposited in the bronchial region rather than in the trachea. Bronchial reactivity was increased by all concentrations of ozone alone. When the two pollutants were combined the resultant joint response was antagonism. Why the combination should reduce the effectiveness of either pollutant alone is unknown.

Rabbits were exposed for 2 hr/day on 5 days/wk for up to a year to 125 $\mu g/m^3$ sulfuric acid, 0.1 ppm ozone and to the combination (Schlesinger et al. 1992b). Some animals were kept for a 6 month post-exposure period. The criteria of response were quantitative and temporal alterations in tracheobronchial mucociliary clearance function and bronchial epithelial secretory cells. Clearance times were altered by exposure to sulfuric acid or to the mixture and became progressively slower following the end of exposure, The ozone alone did not alter clearance during exposure, but the rate slowed during the post exposure observation period. There was no evidence of synergism or antagonism on clearance rates. Histological examination of the intrapulmonary conducting airways was done after 4, 8 or 12 months of exposure and after the post-exposure period. Sulfuric acid produced an increase in the number of secretory cells in small airways by 12 months of exposure. Ozone and the mixture produced an increase in secretory cell number by 4 months, but the response became attenuated with continued exposure. There was evidence of synergism between ozone and acid at 4 months and antagonism at subsequent times. These studies are relevant because the ozone level was below the current Federal standard and the sulfuric acid level was not far above measured peaks. The complex nature of pollutant interactions is shown clearly by the finding of both synergism and antagonism that seemed to depend upon the duration of exposure. More long-term exposure studies using a variety of criteria are vital to an understanding of these important phenomena.

Particulate Sulfite: The Neglected Pollutant?

As was discussed above, metal oxide aerosols with sorbed sulfuric acid occur in the atmosphere. Stable S^{IV} aerosols have been found in plumes and effluents from power plants and smelters (Eatough et al. 1980, 1981,

DasGupta 1982). The concentrations of these particulate sulfite species were approximately 10 to 30% of the total suspended sulfur oxide aerosols. Sulfite aerosols have also been observed in the ambient air of California (Novakov et al. 1972). In our preliminary studies of the effect of various mixing conditions on the interaction of sulfur dioxide and zinc oxide we found that when the two were mixed at ambient temperatures in the presence of water vapor the predominant particulate sulfur species formed was S^{IV} as indicated by ESCA analysis and later confirmed quantitatively by ion chromatography. Although we were not able, because of limited personnel and the higher priority of sulfuric acid sorbed particles, to pursue the examination of the pulmonary response to these sulfite aerosols, we did observe that a 1-hour exposure of guinea pigs to 1 mg/m^3 zinc oxide plus 1 ppm sulfur dioxide mixed under these conditions produced an increase in airway resistance of 29% and a decrease in compliance of 13% as measured by the Amdur-Mead method (Amdur et al. 1983). The resistance increase, unlike that produced by sulfuric acid-sorbed particles, was reversible by 1 hour post-exposure but the compliance decrease persisted. If one accepts the Amdur-Mead method as predictive of the response of asthmatics, these data suggest that the sulfite aerosols could be of importance.

Exposure of guinea pigs for 1 hour to aerosols of sodium sulfite with mass mean diameter (MMD) of 0.36 μm at concentrations of 474, 669 or 972 μg sulfite/m^3 caused dose related increases in airway resistance and decreases in compliance (Chen et al. 1987). When calculated as resistance change per μmol of S/m^3 the sodium sulfite was a less potent irritant than sulfuric acid of the same particle size. Animals were also exposed for 1 hour to 204, 395 and 1152 μg/m^3 sulfite and compartments of lung volume, DL_{CO} and wet lung weight/body weight ratio were measured. Dose-related decreases in lung volumes and DL_{CO} and increases in wet lung/body weight were observed. When the data for 395 μg/m^3 (3 μmol/m^3) are compared with the response to 390 μg/m^3 (4 μmol/m^3) sulfuric acid of the same particle size the sulfite produced statistically significant decreases in all compartments of lung volume and DL_{CO} whereas the sulfuric acid produced no change in the 1-hour exposure. This is an interesting and perhaps somewhat unexpected finding. It makes it even more regrettable that data are not available on the effects of sulfite-sorbed zinc oxide on these respiratory parameters.

Last et al. (1980) found that in rats exposed continuously for 3 days to 1, 6 and 14 mg/m^3 sodium sulfite a statistically significant dose-related increase in lung wet to dry weight ratio was seen. Exposure to 100 μg/m^3

showed a non-significant trend towards such an increase. These changes are indicative of pulmonary edema and/or inflammation. Sodium sulfite aerosols also caused an increased glycoprotein secretion in rat tracheo-explants.

Recently Heyder's (1992) group in Germany did extensive and meticulous studies of the respiratory response of beagle dogs exposed for 290 days to respirable sulfite aerosol at a concentration of 300 µg/m³. One might wish that all such chronic studies were so thoughtfully planned. Functional pulmonary response was assessed by measuring respiratory lung functions, examining lung lavage fluid, and by studying clearance of radiolabeled test particles from the lung periphery. The structural responses of the airways and peripheral airspaces were studied by semiquantitative morphology and quantitative morphometry using light, scanning and transmission electron microscopy.

Respiratory lung function tests were done at the end of the exposure period. The only changes observed were a reduction in lung compliance and a reduction in pulmonary diffusing capacity. The change in diffusing capacity correlated with a decrease in alveolar surface area as demonstrated by postmortem morphometric analysis. Bronchoalveolar lavage (BAL) was performed every 7 weeks. Protein and albumin concentrations in BAL fluid increased during the second half of exposure, indicating leakage of serum proteins into the alveolar lumen. The relative levels of methionine sulfoxide and carbonyl groups in the BAL protein, indicators for oxidative reactions in the respiratory tract, were lowered at the start of exposure. This indicates either a lowered oxidant burden and/or an increased antioxidant capacity in the lungs. In addition there was increased release of the lysosomal enzyme b-N-acetylglocosaminidase from phagocytes. The increased enzyme activity combined with increased protein content may indicate participation of leucocytes in the enhanced leakage of protein into the lungs. The number of macrophages did not change during exposure but the numbers of eosinophils and lymphocytes were elevated late. This may be a first indication of allergic and immunological reactions to the exposure. Alveolar macrophages showed a reduced phagocytic capacity and reduced production of oxygen-derived free radicals, indicating an impaired bacterial defense capacity. The *in vivo* translocation rate of moderately soluble particles (Co_3O_4) was increased indicating an enhancement of clearance of these particles from the lung periphery. These results were supported by the greater dissolution of these particles *in vitro* by alveolar macrophages in BAL. Clearance of insoluble fused aluminosilicate particles by mechanical transport from the periphery of the lung was also altered but some dogs showed acceleration and others a retardation of clearance. Postmortem morphologic examination of the respiratory system showed hyperplastic changes in the nasal cavity and disturbance of ciliated cell development in the trachea as well as the decrease in alveolar surface area noted above. This indicates that the entire respiratory tract is susceptible to airborne S^{IV}.

Although the sulfite aerosols have not been as extensively studied as sulfuric acid, the impact of the studies available is not minor. If we accept the fact that in the overall area of the health effects of sulfur aerosols animal work has been a good predictor of the response of human subjects and the results of epidemiology, it would be the path of unwisdom to ignore these studies in assessing health effects in areas where sulfite aerosols have been shown to occur.

Recent Toxicological Studies of Particles

Recent reports (discussed in other chapters) suggesting an association of increased mortality and morbidity with exposure to low levels of PM$_{10}$ at or below the current standards have caused an escalation in toxicological research on particles and been the stimulus for several meetings and symposia at national meetings such as the Society of Toxicology and American Thoracic Society addressing the overall aspects of the problem. Some questions being examined in these studies, namely ultrafine particles and the importance of transition metals in terms of toxicity and non-uniform distribution across particle size are not new and have been shown by the relatively few studies over the last thirty years that directly addressed them to be of great importance. Another question being addressed in these studies is the effect of particles on animal models of human disease such as chronic bronchitis, emphysema, inflammation and pulmonary hypertension. This section will discuss a few of these studies although many of them are available at present only as peer reviewed abstracts rather than complete articles.

A number of these recent studies have utilized collected particles which are then given by intratracheal instillation. It is encouraging that the relationship of biological response and particulate chemical composition, including variations of composition related to particle size, is the focus of these studies. *This, and only this, is the path to eventual understanding of the health effects of air pollution.* Intratracheal instillation has been widely used as a simple means of exposure as it does not involve the complex equipment, expertise and expense involved in inhalation exposure. It is entirely appropriate as the method of necessity to provide needed information on pulmonary toxicity when, as in these studies, only small quantities of collected aerosols are available. Useful toxicological information can be obtained on the effects of a single dose of known quantity. It must, however, be kept firmly in mind that intratracheal instillation is by no means the equivalent of inhalation. The particles reach the lung suspended in saline rather than as airborne particles deposited in specific areas of the lung depending on particle size. Soluble materials sorbed on the surface of a particle could be delivered dissolved in the saline rather than with the deposited particle to produce a high local concentration as would occur in inhalation.

A few recent studies have utilized a particle concentrator (Sioutas et al., 1995) to expose normal and impaired animals by inhalation to enhanced concentrations of ambient particles. This has the advantage that the particles inhaled are those that actually occur in the ambient air. The technique is quite new so there are not yet extensive published studies. It is to be hoped that they too in time will include detailed chemical analysis of the ambient particles, with some emphasis on concentration of critical metals, which would allow possible correlation of biological effects with chemical composition. Without this information one could only conclude that particulate air pollution *per se* is harmful for chronic bronchitic rats as we already know it is for human chronic bronchitics. Results of some of the studies of metals discussed below could provide guidance for selecting atmospheres to be studied. It is also perhaps worth pointing out that as a species rats are quite insensitive to sulfuric acid, a critical component of air pollution, a fact that was established in the early 1950s and extensively re-documented twenty years later.

The current active interest in research on pulmonary effects of ultrafine (below 0.1 μm) particles is both appropriate and overdue. As early as 1935, a physicist made a model of pulmonary deposition that predicted that 68% of inhaled particles 0.03 μm would be deposited (Findeisen, 1935). The model was simplistic and contained some erroneous assumptions about pulmonary anatomy and airflow in the respiratory tract. One respiratory physiologist colleague suggested that Findeisen must have obtained his ideas on the lung from a drunken medical student in a beer hall. Nonetheless, the suggestion that ultrafine particles had potential toxicological importance was in the physiological literature sixty years ago. Subsequent studies on the deposition of 0.04 μm NaCl particles in dogs indicated 66% deposition (Morrow and Gibb, 1958), a value reasonably close to Findeisen's prediction. The most recent International Commission on Radiological Protection (1994) human lung deposition model predicts that 0.02 μm particles have a 50% deposition efficiency in the alveolar region.

Ultrafine particles are emitted into the atmosphere by combustion processes including burning of coal and oil, smelting of metals as well as being present in diesel exhaust and in the exhaust of automobiles equipped with catalytic converters. Although only a small fraction of mass concentration, ultrafine particles are present in large numbers and have a very large surface area. Laboratory studies of the metals present in the ultrafine fraction of aerosols resulting from controlled coal combustion correlated with field studies indicating an enrichment of a variety of metals of toxicological importance in the ultrafine fraction (Quann et al., 1982).

The ability of a freshly formed fume of ultrafine particles of ZnO to produce symptoms of metal fume fever has long been known. When the fume ages the particle size increases by aggregation and the potency is lost. Studies discussed earlier in this chapter indicated that ultrafine ZnO particles with sorbed sulfuric acid were capable of producing functional and pathological alterations in the lungs of guinea pigs as was the ultrafine fraction of coal combustion aerosols.

Ultrafine particles of TiO_2 caused an inflammatory response in alveoli and interstitium of rat lungs that was greater than that observed with 0.2 μm particles. (Öberdorster et al., 1992). The 0.02 μm particles also induced greater cytocine release by alveolar macrophages (Driscoll et al., 1994). Although the TiO_2 particles were individually 0.02 μm they were present in the inhalation chamber as aggregates and thus not inhaled as individual particles. Although these studies made clear the greater potency of the ultrafine particles, the effects were not acute and did not include acute mortality. Concentrations used were high, in the 20 mg/m^3 range.

More recently Öberdorster et al. (1995) exposed rats to fume of thermodegredation products of polytetrafluoroethylene (Teflon) which were present as singlet particles of 0.02 μm. Up to a temperature of 405^0 C minimal particles were produced. The particle number increased dramatically as the temperature was increased reaching a concentration of about 1 x 10^6 particles/cm^3 when the furnace temperature reached 425° C. Rats were exposed for 30 min. The lungs were lavaged 4 hours after exposure. No inflammatory response was produced by the lowest furnace temperature. At 420°C inflammation was present with 85% of the lavagable cells polymorphonuclear leucocytes. Lavage protein was increased by a factor of 10 over control values. At the highest temperature none of the animals survived to the 4-hour time point. The lavage fluid was bloody and the lungs showed evidence of acute hemorrhagic inflammatory edema. The furnace temperature was below that needed to produce the highly toxic vapor phase compounds associated with thermal degradation of Teflon, so the observed pulmonary response could be attributed to the ultrafine fume particles.

The authors appear to attribute the greater toxicity of these particles as compared with the TiO_2 they studied earlier primarily to the fact that they were inhaled as singlet particles of 0.02 μm rather than as aggregates. It is indeed well known that the toxicity of polymer fume, as with zinc fume, is reduced when aggregates form on aging. It has been established that ultrafine particles interact directly with the alveolar epithelium and, as with extremely fine asbestos fibers, translocate readily into the pulmonary interstitium. Such particles can also affect the endothelial cells and cause severe damage to the integrity of both epithelial and endothelial cell layers of the alveoli. Because these ultrafine particles are deposited in substantial amounts in the alveoli their potential for causing damage to the peripheral areas of the lung is obviously very great. The authors state that ambient ultrafine particles are inhaled as singlet particles although they do not document this statement.

That their concentration of particles is relevant to levels occurring in urban areas is supported by measurements cited by Öberdoster et al. that were made in 1993 in Bologna, Italy that found concentrations of particles 0.02–0.05 μm up to 2.4×10^5 particles/cm^3. The concentration of 1×10^6 particles/cm^3 in their exposures was only four times this level so the concentration used was realistic. If the experimental results were indeed accounted for primarily on the basis of particle size rather than on the intrinsic chemical toxicity of the fume, a factor of four seems a slim margin indeed between lethal pulmonary effects in healthy rats exposed for 30 min and no serious illness among the citizens of Bologna inhaling particles of the same size. Such highly toxic aerosols produced by thermal degradation of teflon are hardly a surrogate for ultrafine ambient aerosols.

Freshly generated ultrafine carbon particles with sorbed sulfuric acid were used to examine the importance of both mass concentration and particle number on irritant response (Chen et al. 1995). This system permitted the mass concentration to be held constant while particle number was varied or the number to be held constant while mass concentration was varied. Guinea pigs were exposed for 3 h to sulfuric acid of 350 μg/m^3 sorbed on 10^6, 10^7, or 10^8 particles/cm^3 and to 50, 100, 200 and 300 μg/m^3 sulfuric acid sorbed on 10^8 particles/cm^3. Alterations in phagocytic capacity, intracellular pH and intracellular free calcium of magrophages harvested 24 h after exposure by bronchoalveolar lavage. At a fixed number concentration there was a sulfuric acid concentration-dependent decrease in phagocytic capacity (PC), pH and calcium. At a fixed mass concentration, 10^8 particles/cm^3 decreased the pH but lower numbers of particles with sorbed acid did not. These results indicate that both the amount of acid sorbed on the ultrafine carbon particles and the numbers of particles are factors in defining the aerosol's irritant potency.

Not surprisingly recent studies are showing that the concentration of transition metals influences the observed toxicity of atmospheric particles and that these factors are non-uniform across particle size. Research on analysis of metals in ambient air samples, including variation of certain metals with particle size, was active twenty years ago (Risby 1979). Many of these metals are sorbed on the surface of particles (Linton et al. 1976). Similar surface enrichment was found in laboratory studies of aerosols from controlled combustion of coals (Amdur et al. 1986). The metal sorbed on the surface rather than the total metal content is important in governing potential toxic response. Recent studies indicate that acid soluble concentrations of first row transition metals which correlate with concentrations of ohmic-acid like materials capable of complexing metals in atmospheric samples (Prichard and Ghio 1995, Ghio et al. 1996). To be toxicologically active, the metals must be bioavailable. Principles determining the bioavailability of particle-adsorbed air pollutants have been recently reviewed by Sehnert, Long and Risby (1996). It will be important to know the form and valence state of the surface sorbed metals.

Samples of PM$_{10}$ from northern Mexico City, the focus of industrial activity, and central and southern areas of the city where motor vehicles, pollen and soil are the main pollution sources were compared as to concentrations of Cu, Ni, V, Zn and Fe and their cytotoxicity to human lung fibroblasts (Osornio-Vargas et al. 1996). Total soluble transition metals were highest in the sample from the northern industrial area which produced a measureable concentration-dependent cytotoxic effect (EC50) of 30µg/m^3 whereas the other two dusts caused negligible cytotoxicity at similar or higher doses. It would be interesting indeed to have inhalation exposure data using the particle concentrator mentioned above on these three atmospheres.

Ambient particles from Washington, DC were collected in size ranges of <1.7 µm, 1.7–3.7 µm and 3.7–20 µm, analyzed for transition metals and given to rats by intratracheal instillation (Dreher et al. 1996). The <1.7 µm fraction had the lowest total transition metal content but the highest percentage of soluble transition metals, the highest sulfate content and was the most acidic of the three size fractions. Bronchoalveolar lavage fluid 24 hours after exposure showed greatest lung injury from the <1.7 μm fraction as indicated by larger increases in protein, albumin, red blood cells and eosinophils. Washing the <1.7 μm particles with water attenuated these effects and a particle-free leachate duplicated the effect of the particles.

Another study (Gavett et al., 1996) compared the ability of two samples of residual oil fly ash (ROFA) to produce pulmonary injury when given to rats by intratracheal instillation. Analysis showed that ROFA-1 had twice as much saline-leachable V, Ni, and sulfate and 40 times as much Fe as ROAF-2. Sample ROAF-2 had a 30-fold higher content of Zn. In rats examined 4 days after instillation baseline pulmonary function parameters and airway hyperreactivity to acetylcholine challenge were significantly worse in the ROAF-2 exposed rats. Neutrophils in BAL and pathological indices were also greater in the ROAF-2. These results re-enforce the possible importance of Zn in producing pulmonary damage. These new results are interesting in the context of historic air pollution related research. In 1955 Hemeon published results of an analysis of a filter from an air conditioner that had been running specifically during the Donora, PA air pollution incident in 1948 (Hemeon, 1955). His analysis showed that 22% of the material was water soluble. Of this water soluble fraction, 58% was zinc ammonium sulfate and 21% was zinc sulfate. Stimulated by these results, Amdur and Corn (1963) exposed guinea pigs to aerosols of these compounds and found that they increased pulmonary flow resistance in a dose-dependent manner and that the irritant potency increased with decreasing particle size over a range of 1.4 to 0.3 μm.

Particles of both natural and anthropogenic origin can include soluble metal salts and also contain metals complexed at the surface of an insoluble particle. Those metals that exist in more than one stable valence state can catalyze an electron transfer and therefore have the capacity to generate oxidants in biological systems. Thus pulmonary effects of exposure to such particles may resemble those produced by an oxidant gas including neutrophilic alveolitis, airway hyperreactivity and increased virulence of pulmonary infection leading to enhanced mortality.

These questions were addressed by Prichard et al. (1996) in a study of the pulmonary response to ten aerosols relative to their content of the first row transition metals: Ti, V, Cr, Mn, Fe, Co, Ni and Cu. The aerosols included desert dust, Mt. Saint Helens volcanic ash, two ambient air samples, four samples of coal fly ash and two samples of oil fly ash. Soluble concentrations of the metals were measured in 1.0 N HCl extracts with inductively coupled plasma emission spectroscopy. The metal in highest concentration was Fe except in the two oil fly ash samples in which V predominated. To assay *in vitro* oxidant, thiobarbituric acid reactive products of deoxyribose were measured following incubation with the sample. The amount of oxidation varied widely among the samples. There was correlation of the oxidation with the content of soluble metals that was statistically significant except for Ti and V. When the hydroxyl radical scavengers dimethylsulfoxide or dimethylthiourea were added to the incubation mixture, chromogen formation was inhibited in a dose dependent manner. In rats the concentration of protein and the percentage of neutrophils in bronchoalveolar lavage fluid collected 96 hours after tracheal instillation of the samples in saline were increased. The magnitude of these increases again correlated with the individual metals.

Three representative samples were chosen for further study: Mt. Saint Helens ash, one of the ambient air samples and an oil fly ash. The concentration of soluble metals was lowest in the volcanic ash, intermediate in the ambient air sample and highest in the oil fly ash. A high percentage of the metal in the oil fly ash was water soluble. Pathologic examination of the lungs of rats 96 hours after instillation showed that the ambient air sample and the oil fly ash produced cell proliferation, inflammation and distortion of the normal alveolar architecture. Particles could be discerned within macrophages. Airway hyperreactivity in rats was measured 96 hours after intratracheal instillation using acetylcholine challenge. The degree of airway hyperreactivity increased with increasing metal content of the three samples. The ambient air sample and the oil fly ash increased mortality to subsequent bacterial challenge in mice.

Recent studies have demonstrated using various animal models of human cardioplumonary disease that impaired animals show increased sensitivity to inhalation of particles as do individuals with pre-existing disease in exposed human populations. Godleski et al. (1996) exposed normal rats and rats with monocrotyline-induced pulmonary inflammation or sulfur dioxide-induced chronic bronchitis concentrated ambient air particles (230–270 µg/m^3) for 6 hours on 3 consecutive days. No mortality occurred in the normal animals but mortality was 19% in the inflammation group and 37% in the chronic bronchitis group. Pathologic examination indicated no inflammation and minimal bronchoconstriction in normal animals. The animals with pre-existing inflammation showed acute inflammation of alveoli and interstitium and some bronchoconstriction. The animals with chronic bronchitis showed airway inflammation, increased mucus, interstitial edema, pulmonary vascular congestion and marked bronchoconstriction. In both the diseased groups bronchoconstriction was significantly greater in the animals that died compared to those that were killed which suggests its possible role in the deaths.

Costa et al. (1995) examined the effect of pulmonary hypertension on the response to Mt. Saint Helens volcanic ash, that had been shown to produce minimal inflammation, and a coal fly ash that had been shown to be highly reactive. Two established rat models of pulmonary hypertension were used: primary pulmonary hypertension due to monocrotaline vascular injury and pulmonary hypertension secondary to elastase-induced pulmonary emphysema. Untreated rats served as controls. Exposure was by intratracheal instillation. At 96 hours post-exposure bronchoalveolar lavage fluid was collected to examine inflammatory markers, total cell and differential counts, Lactic dehydrogenaze (LDH), protein and Thio Barbitonic Acid (TBA) reactive products which provide evidence of nonspecific oxidation. The rats with emphysema showed only slight increases in inflammatory markers compared to untreated rats while the monocrotaline treated rats had increases in protein (15X) and LDH (5X) without an increase in cells. The emphysemic rats showed minimal enhancement of the particulate effects, probably due to the moderate level of disease. The monocrotaline-treated rats had one death in the Mt. Saint Helens group and two in the coal fly ash group. The Mt. Saint Helens ash produced no greater inflammation than the monocrotaline alone but the inflammatory markers were markedly increased in the coal fly ash exposed group. These data suggest that pulmonary hypertension may be a risk factor in exposure to ambient aerosols that produce an inflammatory response.

Summary

The results of toxicological studies on experimental animals provide part of the data base used to evaluate the health effects of air pollutants. It is therefore of importance to examine how well the animal data have predicted the response of human subjects. If such studies are to be usefully predictive, toxicologists must use criteria that are both sensitive and biologically relevant to responses of people exposed to pollution. *Extrapolation from results obtained on high concentrations is not appropriate.*

Data are presented on the comparative toxicity of sulfur dioxide and sulfuric acid. The animal data obtained by measurement of airway resistance in guinea pigs and of bronchial clearance of particles in donkeys predicted clearly that sulfuric acid was more irritant than sulfur dioxide. Data obtained on human subjects confirmed this prediction. These acute studies also correctly predicted the comparative toxicity of the two compounds in two year studies of monkeys. Such chronic studies are not possible in human subjects but it is a reasonable to assume that sulfuric acid would be more toxic than sulfur dioxide. Current findings in epidemiological studies certainly support this assumption.

When levels of pollution rise, the individuals most affected are those with pre-existing cardiopulmonary disease. This was, of course, well documented in the various acute air pollution incidents. Current studies of hospital admissions of patients with respiratory disease show an increase related to pollution levels.

Examination of control and exposure data for about a thousand guinea pigs exposed to a variety of irritant gases or aerosols or to combinations of an inert aerosol with an irritant gas provided an animal analog. Among the total number of animals about 13% showed higher than normal airway resistance. Considered as a group these animals showed a greater than normal increase in airway resistance. When divided according to level of exposure, a higher than normal increase was seen in animals exposed to irritant aerosols or irritant gases plus inert aerosol but not to irritant gases alone. When divided according to degree of response, a higher than normal response was seen in groups with low exposure but the response to large exposures was similar in both high control resistance and normal animals. The ten animals with the highest control airway resistance showed a response twice that of the corresponding normal animals. Three of these animals had received low exposures that produced only a slight response; but this slight response was four to ten times the response of the normal animals with the same exposure. They provide an animal analog of the individuals most affected by increases in air pollution.

In the 1980s data became available indicating that asthmatics responded with an increase in airway resistance at concentrations of sulfur dioxide much lower than those needed to produce a response in normal subjects. The Amdur-Mead guinea pig model that measures increases in airway resistance had predicted this response quantitatively. When data later became available indicating that asthmatic subjects were also more sensitive to sulfuric acid than normal subjects, the animal model had once again been predictive.

Acute studies of bronchomucociliary clearance of particles in both donkeys and rabbits exposed to sulfuric acid have been predictive of the effects of sulfuric acid on particle clearance measured in human subjects. In acute studies of bronchomucociliary clearance the effect of exposure to sulfuric acid and to cigarette smoke are similar in donkeys and human subjects. In both acute and chronic studies in donkeys, the effect of sulfuric acid and of cigarette smoke are similar. In heavy smokers clearance of particles from the bronchial region is seriously impaired. Chronic studies of human subjects to sulfuric acid are neither possible nor ethical. The assumption that the animal model correctly predicts the human response is entirely reasonable. Chronic exposure of rabbits to sulfuric acid produced changes not only in particle clearance but also in a variety of sensitive criteria carefully chosen to be relevant to changes produced by chronic bronchitis and asthma. It is also a reasonable assumption that these results are predictive of the potential effects of sulfuric acid on exposed populations. Recent epidemiology studies seem to suggest that this is so.

If toxicological studies are to be usefully predictive, they must examine not only low concentrations but also specific types of particles known to occur. Field studies have shown that some of the sulfuric acid in the atmosphere is present sorbed on ultrafine metal oxides. These acidic particles are released as primary emissions from smelting operations and coal combustion. Freshly formed aerosols must be used to examine the response to such particles. Collected and resuspended fly ash would be *completely useless* because the sorbed sulfuric acid would not survive such treatment. Sulfuric acid sorbed on ultrafine zinc oxide was used as a prototype aerosol to study the response of guinea pigs. The toxicological criteria were chosen to examine mainly effects in the alveolar regions of the lung where such particles are deposited. A single 3-hour exposure to 30 $\mu g/m^3$ or greater of sorbed sulfuric acid produced dose-related decreases in compartments of lung volume and DL_{CO}. At a concentration of 60 $\mu g/m^3$ these changes as well as increases in cell count, protein and various enzymes in bronchoalveolar lavage fluid were only slowly reversible. Pathological examination indicated damage to the centriacinar region of the lung and evidence of pulmonary edema. Repeated 5 day exposures to 20 or 30 $\mu g/m^3$ sorbed sulfuric acid produced changes that were dose-related, progressive and related to the cumulative dose (concentration x time). These exposures also made the lung more sensitive to reexposure to sorbed sulfuric acid and also to ozone exposure. The sorbed sulfuric acid was a more potent irritant than free sulfuric acid of the same size. No data are available on the response of human subjects to these aerosols, but it is my educated guess that the response in guinea pigs is predictive of that response.

During combustion of certain coals as much as 9% of the sulfur in the coal is emitted as sulfuric acid sorbed on the ultrafine fraction of the ash. Analytical chemistry studies showed that the ultrafine ash from combustion of Illinois No. 6 coal carried sorbed sulfuric acid and that the ultrafine ash from Montana Lignite, a more alkaline coal, carried sorbed neutralized sulfate. The acidic ash from Illinois No. 6 produced pulmonary alterations similar to those produced by the sulfuric acid sorbed on zinc oxide. These changes were not observed following exposure to the neutral ash of Montana Lignite. It is possible that sulfuric acid sorbed on ultrafine fly ash could have been a contributing factor in the increased incidence of wheeze noted a population living down stream from a coal burning power plant in the Chestnut Ridge area of Pennsylvania.

The potential for joint toxic action of ozone and sulfuric acid is of considerable importance and is under active investigation. Studies of hospital admissions for respiratory related disorders and studies of pulmonary function in children attending summer camps strongly suggest that the presence of both pollutants is an important determinant of the observed responses. Extensive studies in the rat, a species sensitive to ozone but quite insensitive to sulfuric acid, have shown that sulfuric acid potentiates the response to ozone as evaluated by sensitive biochemical criteria of lung damage such as increased protein content or apparent increased collagen synthesis. Morphological studies showed that ultrafine (0.03 μm) sulfuric acid potentiated the response to ozone but fine (0.3 μm) sulfuric acid did not. Recent acute and chronic studies of rabbits using criteria such as particle clearance, macrophage function and sensitivity of the lung to acetylcholine challenge have produced mixed results. Sometime potentiation is seen, whereas other times antagonism results. Obviously further research is needed to clarify this important problem.

Stable sulfite aerosols have been found in plumes and effluents from power plants and smelters in concentrations of 10 to 30% of the total suspended sulfur oxide aerosols. Such aerosols have also been detected in the ambient air of California. Guinea pigs exposed for 1 hour to sodium sulfite aerosols from 200 to 1000 μg/m^3 showed a dose-related responses. These included increases in airway resistance and wet lung/body weight ratios and decreases in compliance, compartments of lung volume and DL$_{CO}$. Exposure of beagle dogs for 290 days to respirable sulfite aerosol at a concentration of 300 μg/m^3 produced a variety of pulmonary changes. Lung compliance and DL$_{CO}$ were reduced, the latter correlating with a decrease in alveolar surface area. Protein and albumin levels in BAL fluid increased. Alveolar macrophages showed a reduced phagocytic capacity and reduced production of oxygen-derived free radicals indicating impaired bacterial defense capacity. Translocation rate of moderately soluble particles increased indicating enhancement of clearance from the lung periphery. Clearance of insoluble particles by mechanical transport from the lung periphery was accelerated in some dogs and retarded in others. Hyperplastic changes in the nasal cavity indicated the entire respiratory tract was susceptible to damage by airborne sulfite.

Unlike sulfate, sulfite has been long known to cause a variety of biological responses. Although the data on pulmonary response to inhaled sulfite aerosols is not extensive, the impact of the studies available is not minor. (Sulfite aerosols could well contribute to observed health effects in situations where they are present in appreciable concentrations.)

Overall the data presented and the correlation with response of human subjects have shown that when the toxicological criteria chosen are sensitive and relevant to human health effects the animal response is predictive of the response in human subjects. When epidemiologists finally paid attention to what the animals were trying to tell them, their results became more definitive (Amdur 1989).

Recent reports suggesting an association of increased mortality and morbidity with exposures to low levels of PM_{10} at or below the current standard have stimulated interest in toxicological research on particles. The pulmonary effects of inhalation of ultrafine particles of TiO_2, sulfuric acid sorbed on carbon particles, and fume from thermodegradation of Teflon have been examined. Ultrafine particles are important because they are present in large numbers and are deposited in the alveolar regions of the lung where their irritant effects are produced. Collected atmospheric particles, Mt. Saint Helens volcanic ash, and samples of coal and oil fly ash have been examined using intratracheal instillation as the route of exposure. Transition metals that exist in more than one stable valence state have the capacity to generate oxidants in biological systems. Pulmonary effects of exposure to such particles may resemble those produced by an oxidant gas including neutrophilic alveolitis, airway hyperreactivity and increased virulence of pulmonary infection leading to enhanced mortality. Observed effects are correlated with the concentration of ionizable and soluble metals of the various aerosols studied but not with total metal content. Many of the transition metals tend to be enriched on the surface of particles. Recent studies have shown using various animal models of human cardiopulmonary disease that impaired animals show increased sensitivity to particulate exposure. Rats with pre-existing inflammation or chronic bronchitis showed evidence of pulmonary damage and bronchial constriction following inhalation of concentrated ambient air particles that were not observed in normal rats. Pulmonary hypertension increased the inflammatory response in rats following intratracheal instillation of coal fly ash suggesting that it may be a risk factor in exposure to ambient aerosols that produce an inflammatory response.

6

Epidemiology of Acute Health Effects: Summary of Time-Series Studies

Douglas Dockery and Arden Pope

Introduction

In this and the following chapter, studies relating mortality and various morbidity outcomes to air pollution are reviewed. An association between human health and air pollution has been proposed for more than 50 years. Over the last 10–15 years air pollution measurements in the U.S., Canada and elsewhere have been vastly improved. The WHO GEMS program has promoted standardized sampling for several air pollutants. Nationalized health care systems in many developed countries have given researchers new opportunities to explore the relationships between pollution and various diagnostic outcomes for both illness and cause of death. Ease of access to electronically archived data has also helped facilitate the proliferation of air pollution and health studies since the mid 1980s.

Nearly all of the currently available epidemiology studies of air pollution fall within two broad classifications of study design which include 1) acute exposure studies which are typically time-series studies and use short-term changes in air pollution over time (usually 1–5 days) as the source of exposure variability and 2) chronic exposure studies which are principally cross-sectional in design and use longer-term pollution data (usually 1 year or more). These studies can also be subdivided into population-based (ecological) studies where the units of comparison are entire populations of communities or neighborhoods, and cohort-based studies in which the unit of comparison for health outcomes and co-risk factors are individuals enrolled in a well-defined cohort or sample (see Figure 6.1). In this Chapter 6, epidemiological studies of acute exposure will be discussed. In Chapter 7 epidemiological studies of "chronic" exposure

FIGURE 6.1

Basic Study Designs of Currently Published Studies of Health Effects of Particulate Air Pollution

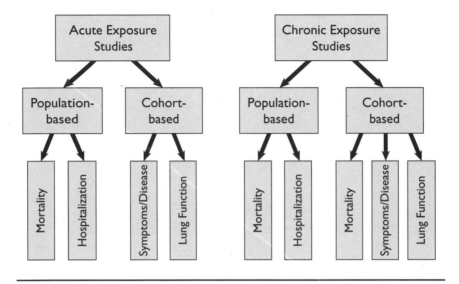

will be discussed, in which the sustained exposure to lower levels of pollutants is related to mortality or morbidity.

Recent studies have observed adverse effects at ambient pollution levels common to many U.S. cities and reflect the results of many people's daily exposure. Much of the evidence has come from studies in the U.S. where ambient air pollution has improved substantially, as indicated by lower levels of SO_2 and total suspended particulate pollution. So these recent studies suggest that adverse health effects are evident at much lower levels than previously thought or some important component(s) of ambient air pollution, such as combustion-source fine particles are not being adequately controlled for with current National Ambient Air Quality Standards.

Studies of air pollution episodes

As mentioned in Chapter 1, early studies focused on severe air pollution episodes, often in narrow industrial valleys such as the Meuse River in Belgium (Firket 1931) and Donora, PA (Ciocco & Thompson 1961). The most dramatic of these documented air pollution episodes occurred in London, England (Logan 1953, Wilkins 1953, Ministry of Health 1954). Several later studies in London reported associations between daily mortality air pollution at much lower pollution levels (Ostro 1984,

Schwartz and Marcus 1990, Ito et al. 1993). Elevated respiratory and cardiovascular disease morbidity and mortality have also been reported for a more moderate increase in pollution in the North Rhine–Westfalia area of Germany (Wichmann et al. 1989).

The severe air pollution episodes have been frequently reviewed (Ellison & Waller 1978, Holland et al. 1979, Shy 1979, Bates 1980). They demonstrated an important link between cardiopulmonary disease mortality and morbidity with extremely elevated concentrations of particulate and/or sulfur oxide air pollution. They also suggested effects at lower levels. Although the biological mechanisms involved were poorly understood, there remained little disagreement that, at very high levels, ambient air pollution can be an important risk factor associated with increased cardiopulmonary disease and early mortality. It is important to recognize that the particle and SO_2 concentrations measured or estimated for these severe acute episodes ranged between 500 $\mu g/m^3$ and almost 2 mg/m^3. These levels are higher than now occur in any U.S. cities, but levels of air pollution in these higher ranges are observed in many developing nations and in parts of Russia and the former soviet block countries.

Health effects at low levels of air pollution

A primary interest with respect to air pollution policy among most developed countries over the last 20 years has been to determine the lowest level, and length of exposure to air pollution that can cause adverse health effects. It has often been assumed that there is a threshold, or safe level, below which there are no substantial health effects. A common public policy approach, therefore, was to attempt to find this safe threshold level and establish goals or standards that would bring the concentration of air pollution below this level. However, over the years with improved air monitoring, improved collection of health data, and improved designs of epidemiological studies, adverse health effects have been linked to air pollution at smaller and smaller concentrations. The results of these studies are often interpreted to suggest either that there is no safe threshold, or if a threshold exists it is below 1996 ambient levels in the U.S. Many of the studies suggest linear, proportional exposure-response relationship, with no threshold. No single epidemiological study can rigorously prove a causal relationship at today's ambient air pollution concentrations. The suggestion of a causal relationship between current ambient air pollution concentrations is based on a large and growing body of research. Numerous time-series studies have observed associations between particulate air pollution and various human health endpoints, including:

■ mortality,

■ hospitalization for respiratory and heart disease,

■ aggravation of asthma,

■ incidence and duration of respiratory symptoms,

■ lung function, and

■ restricted activity.

The analysis of the relationship between air pollution and health end-points in early studies of severe pollution episodes could rely on relatively simple comparative statistics. The observed associations were often so pronounced that the temporal associations could be easily observed without the use of formal time-series statistical analysis. Recent epidemiologic studies are designed to quantify of more subtle health effects associated with much smaller day-to-day changes in air pollution. Most of these recent studies that have evaluated the health effects of acute or short-term exposure to air pollution, therefore, have required the use of contemporary time-series statistical analysis techniques or related types of analysis. This chapter will first discuss the studies that evaluated the effects of acute pollution exposure on mortality and then those that evaluated the effects of acute pollution exposure on morbidity.

Acute Mortality

Daily time-series mortality studies

A series of recent studies analyzed the temporal distribution of deaths and particulate air pollution at current levels. The U.S. EPA has reviewed these studies in the recent criteria document on the health affects of particulate air pollution and other reviews of these studies have been made (Ostro 1993, Schwartz 1994e, Dockery & Pope 1994, Pope et al. 1995b). These studies observed changes in daily death counts associated with short-term changes in particulate air pollution. A particulate pollution threshold was not generally observed in these studies. The relative risk of mortality increased monotonically with particulate concentrations—usually in a near linear fashion. Table 6.1 summarizes daily time-series studies that have been conducted in the last decade. Figures 6.2 and 6.3 illustrate the variation between several of them graphically. These studies have observed similar particulate air pollution effects in varied locations.

Because various measurements of particulate pollution were used, precise comparisons between studies are difficult. But when particulate mea-

T A B L E   6 . 1
Summary of Selected Acute (Daily Time Series) Mortality Studies

Study area and period	Reference	Particulate Measure	Mean[a] PM$_{10}$ (µg/m³)	Percent Increase in Mortality per 10 µg/m³ Increase in PM$_{10}$ (95% CI)		
				Total	Respiratory	Cardiovascular
Santa Clara, CA 1980–82, 1984–86	Fairley (1990)	Coefficient of Haze	35	0.8 (0.2, 1.5)	3.5 (1.5, 5.6)	0.8 (0.1, 1.6)
Philadelphia, PA 1973–80	Schwartz & Dockery (1992a)	TSP (2-day mean)	40	1.2 (0.7, 1.7)	3.3 (0.1, 6.6)	1.7 (1.0, 2.4)
Utah Valley, UT 1985–89	Pope, et al. (1992)	PM$_{10}$ (5-day mean)	47	1.5 (0.9, 2.1)	3.7 (0.7, 6.7)	1.8 (0.4, 3.3)
Birmingham, AL 1985–88	Schwartz (1993a)	PM$_{10}$ (3-day mean)	48	1.0 (0.2, 1.9)	1.5 (-5.8, 9.4)	1.6 (-0.5, 3.7)
Cincinnati, OH 1977–82	Schwartz (1994f)	TSP	42	1.1 (0.5, 1.7)	2.7 (-0.9, 6.6)	1.4 (0.5, 2.4)
St. Louis, MO 1985–86	Dockery et al. (1992)	PM$_{10}$ (prev. day)	28	1.5 (0.1, 2.9)	NA	NA
Kingston, TN 1985–86	Dockery et al. (1992)	PM$_{10}$ (prev. day)	30	1.6 (-1.3, 4.6)	NA	NA
Detroit, MI 1973–82	Schwartz (1991)	TSP	48	1.0 (0.5, 1.6)	NA	NA
Steubenville, OH 1974–84	Schwartz & Dockery (1992b)	TSP	61	0.7 (0.4, 1.0)	NA	NA
Athens, Greece	Touloumi et al. (1994)	Smoke	NA	0.9 (0.7, 1.2)	NA	NA
Los Angeles, CA	Kinney et al. (1995)	PM$_{10}$	58	0.5 (0.0, 1.1)	NA	NA
Santiago, Chile	Ostro et al. (1995)	PM$_{10}$	115	0.6 (0.4, 0.9)	NA	NA
Chicago, USA	Ito et al. (1995)	PM$_{10}$	NA	0.5 (0.1, 1.0)	NA	NA
Amsterdam, NL	Verhoeff et al. (1996)	PM$_{10}$	NA	0.6 (-0.1, 1.4)	NA	NA
Erfurt, Germany 1988–89	Spix et al. (1994)	SP(same day)	NA	0.6 (0.1, 1.1)	NA	NA
Sao Paulo, Brazil 1990–1991	Saldiva et al. (1995)	PM$_{10}$ (2-day mean)	82	1.3[b] (0.7, 1.9)	NA	NA

a Conversions to PM$_{10}$ assumed that PM$_{10}$ = 0.55xTSP; PM$_{10}$ = CoH/0.55 and PM$_{10}$ = 0.9 smoke (for more detail on the calculations see Dockery and Pope, 1994).

b In the Sao Paulo study mortality counts were only for the elderly (65+ years of age).

Source: Updated from Dockery and Pope (1994).

FIGURE 6.2

Estimated Mean Daily (Oral) Mortality Effects (with 95th Confidence Intervals) for an Increase of 10 μg/m³ PM₁₀

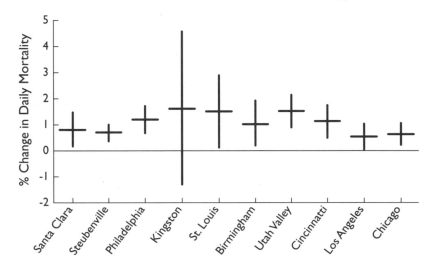

FIGURE 6.3

Estimated Mean Daily Specific Mortality Effects (with 95th Percentile Confidence Intervals) for an Increase of 10 μg/m³ PM₁₀

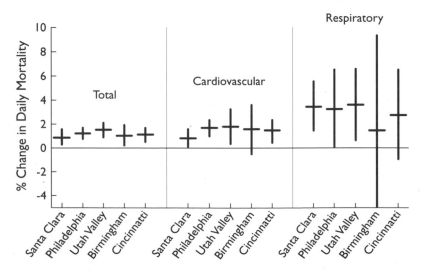

surements are converted to PM_{10} (for more detail on conversions see Dockery and Pope, 1994), there is remarkable consistency in the estimated effect of PM_{10} across these studies. All but one of the studies shows a statistically significant effect, and the estimate of that effect ranges between a 0.5 percent and 1.6 percent in daily mortality for each 10 $\mu g/m^3$ increase in PM_{10} concentration with a weighted mean of about 0.8 percent.

Five of these studies also provided a breakdown of mortality by broad cause-of-death categories. Particulate air pollution generally had the largest effect on respiratory disease mortality but effects on cardiovascular mortality were also observed. An examination of cardiovascular deaths in Philadelphia reported that on days with high particulate air pollution there was a substantial increase in respiratory factors as contributing causes for death, with cardiovascular disease reported as the underlying cause of death (Schwartz 1994c).

For several of these cities, the data have been reanalyzed by Samet, Zeger and Berhane (1995) with results similar to those of the original authors. These reanalysts conclude that their "report lays to rest (the idea) that the originally reported associations between particulate air pollution and increased mortality may have been spurious in some sense."

Shape of the mortality exposure-response relationship and lead-lag relationships

Most of the recent daily time-series mortality studies evaluated the shape of the exposure-response relationship and explored for a safe threshold level. This was typically done by introducing quintile or quartile indicator variables in the regression models or by nonparametric smoothing. Both of these approaches allow for possible nonlinear relationships and, if a threshold exists within the range of pollution studied, would potentially allow for the observation of a threshold level. The PM_{10} values varied in a typical U.S. city from 10 to 120 $\mu g/m^3$ and as high as 365 $\mu g/m^3$ in the Utah Valley.

In general, the estimated exposure-response relationships between daily mortality and air pollution were not consistent with a simple threshold model. It was commonly observed that an exposure-response relationship was consistently monatonic across the range of particulate air pollution concentrations. The shape of this relationship was typically near linear (or log-linear). These results suggest three possibilities: (1) no threshold exists; (2) the threshold is below existing pollution levels that have been studied; or (3) data and methodological constraints result in the estimated relationship looking more linear than it really is. The fact that daily time-series mortality studies consistently observe a positive association between particulate air pollution and daily mortality but do not reveal some lower level at which no effects are observed remains a troubling observation.

Many of the recent daily time-series mortality studies also observe a lead-lag relationship between air pollution and mortality. It would violate a basic tenet of causality if the observed mortality effect predated the exposure. The results of most of the studies indicated that the increased mortality occurred concurrently or within 1–5 days following an increase in air pollution.

As noted in the introduction, an important issue is the extent to which the prompt mortality is reducing life expectancy. Were the people whose deaths are attributed to air pollution about to die within a few days anyway (an effect often referred to as "harvesting")? If so, the Loss of Life Expectancy (LOLE) is the mortality rate multiplied by a small fraction of a year. Or are they people who might have lived several more years? In which case the Loss of Life Expectancy (LOLE) is many times larger.

In the time series studies, the "harvesting" effect would show up as a delayed *negative* correlation of mortality with air pollution variables. This was not seen in the London 1952 air pollution incident, and would be difficult to see if spread out over more than a month. Studies in the next chapter provide evidence of substantial loss of life due to chronic exposure.

Acute Morbidity

The reliable studies in environmental health are mortality studies. That is because mortality is a very objective health end point, whereas morbidity is often less so. This makes mortality studies easier and more free of bias than morbidity studies. Nonetheless, if daily mortality is associated with daily particulate pollution levels, then associations with morbidity should also be observed. Bates (1992) has noted that compelling evidence of health effects of air pollution would require that adverse effects of air pollution be observable across a range of related health outcomes. As the pollution level gets worse—in a given incident or over a period of time—an individual might develop increased symptoms, lower lung function, need increased medication use, and, ultimately, require higher use of health services. Morbidity effects may help explain the patterns of mortality that have been observed in air pollution studies, as well as being matters of concern themselves. In fact, associations with acute exposure to particulate air pollution have also been observed for various morbidity health endpoints, including increased health care visits for respiratory illness, exacerbations of asthma, increased incidence and duration of respiratory symptoms, and declines in measures of lung function. A brief summary of selected acute morbidity studies is given in Table 6.2.

Hospital usage

Pope (1989) reported the results of a unique natural experiment that occurred in the Utah Valley. During the winter of 1986–1987 a labor dispute resulted in the closure of the local steel mill, the largest single source of particulate air pollution in the valley. During this winter, PM_{10} concentrations averaged 51 μg/m^3 with a high of 113 μg/m^3 compared with a mean of 90 μg/m^3 with a high of 365 μg/m^3 during the previous winter. During this winter, children's hospital admissions for respiratory disease dropped by more than 50 percent, compared with adjacent years. Regression analysis estimated a 4.2 percent increase in asthma and bronchitis admissions of children associated with a 10 μg/m^3 increase in 2-month mean PM_{10}.

In response to this study, Lamm et al. (1994) contended that the drop in hospital admissions was not associated with the closure of the steel mill but rather due to biannual epidemics of respiratory syncytial virus (RSV) that coincidentally occurred during winters when the steel mill was open, but not when it was closed. They supported this position by noting that RSV is correlated with pediatric respiratory admissions and showing that when RSV activity is controlled for in statistical regression models the association between PM_{10} and respiratory hospitalizations is attenuated. The Lamm et al. analysis, however, was deficient because adequate data for regional or local RSV activity was not available. The RSV activity variable used in the analysis was actually pediatric bronchiolitis admissions, an important subset of respiratory admissions.

Pope (1991) had also conducted a follow-up study using the same study period and hospital admissions data set that was used by Lamm et al.. Pope noted that there were relatively few diagnoses where the specific agent of disease was specified. For example, there were only 6 hospitalizations for diagnosed cases of pneumonia due to RSV in Utah Valley during the entire study period. Nevertheless, this study observed that bronchitis, bronchiolitis, asthma and related respiratory admissions for preschool aged children were more than twice as high in Utah Valley during periods when the mill was operating versus when it was closed. If this association was strictly spurious, due to regional epidemics of contagious respiratory disease such as RSV that were coincidentally correlated with the operation of the steel mill, similar associations should be observed in neighboring

TABLE   6.2

Summary of Selected Acute (Daily Time Series) Morbidity Studies of Hospital Usage

Usage Measure	Location	Reference	Measure	% increase in morbidity per 10µg/m³ increase in PM_{10} (95% CI)
Asthma	New York City; Buffalo	Thurston et al. (1992)	SO_4	1.9 (0.4, 3.4) 2.1 (-0.6, 5.0)
	Toronto, Ontario	Thurston et al. (1993)	$PM_{2.5}$	2.1 (-0.8, 5.1)
	Detroit, MI	Schwartz (1994)	PM_{10}	0.5 (-3.3, 4.4)
	Southern Ontario	Burnett et al. (1995)	SO_4	1.0 (0.4, 1.6)
Pneumonia	Birmingham, AL	Schwartz (1994a)	PM_{10}	1.8 (0.7, 2.8)
	Detroit, MI	Schwartz (1994g)	PM_{10}	1.2 (0.4, 1.9)
	Minneapolis/ St. Paul, MN	Schwartz (1994d)	PM_{10}	1.6 (-0.3, 2.9)
COPD	Birmingham, AL	Schwartz (1993)	PM_{10}	2.5 (0.3, 4.7)
	Detroit, MI	Schwartz (1994)	PM_{10}	2.0 (0.9, 3.2)
	Minneapolis/ St. Paul, MN	Schwartz (1994)	PM_{10}	4.6 (1.8, 7.5)
	Southern Ontario	Burnett et al. (1995)	PM_{10}	1.5 (0.8, 2.2)
	Santiago, Chile	Ostro et al. (1995)	PM_{10}	0.6 (0.4, 0.9)
All Respiratory	New York City; Buffalo	Thurston et al.(1992)	SO_4	1.0 (0.2, 1.8) 2.2 (0.6, 3.8)
	Toronto, Ontario	Thurston et al. (1993)	SO_4	3.4 (0.4, 6.4)
	Southern Ontario	Burnett et al. (1994)	SO_4	0.8 (0.4, 1.1)
Coronary Artery Disease	Detroit, MI	Schwartz (1994g)	PM_{10}	0.6 (0.2, 0.9)
	Southern Ontario	Burnett et al. (1995)	SO_4	0.7 (0.2, 1.2)
Dysrythmias	Southern Ontario	Burnett et al. (1995)	SO_4	0.4 (-0.6, 1.4)
	Detroit, MI	Schwartz (1994g)	PM_{10}	0.6 (-0.1, 1.3)
Congestive Heart Failure	Southern Ontario	Burnett et al. (1995)	SO_4	0.9 (0.2, 1.7)
	Detroit, MI	Schwartz (1994g)	PM_{10}	1.0 (0.4, 1.6)

Emergency Department Visits

Asthma	Seattle, WA	Schwartz et al. (1993)	PM_{10} (daily mean)	3.4 (0.9, 6.0)
Respiratory Disease	Steubenville	Samet (1981)	TSP (daily mean)	0.5 (0.0, 1.0)
COPD	Barcelona Spain	Sunyer (1993)	British Smoke	2.3 (1.4, 3.2)

Source: Updated from Dockery and Pope 1994.

communities unaffected by the mill's pollution. No such associations were observed in the neighboring communities in Salt Lake and Cache Valleys. Regression results for Utah and Salt Lake Valleys and "control" regressions in the much less polluted Cache Valley provided no evidence that the correlations between PM_{10} and respiratory admissions were confounded by the bi-annual epidemics.

These results do not suggest that biological agents do not play an important role in respiratory illness and hospitalization. They do suggest that exposure to PM_{10} may make individuals more susceptible to respiratory infection and may contribute to the exacerbation of existing respiratory illness primarily caused by biological agents.

Several studies have found that increased rates of respiratory hospital admissions in southern Ontario are associated with increased sulfate and ozone concentrations (Bates and Sizto 1987, 1989; Burnett et al. 1994). Burnett et al. (1995) also evaluated hospital admissions data for 168 hospitals in Ontario and observed significant positive associations between respiratory and cardiac hospital admissions and sulfate concentrations. Thurston and colleagues have reported similar associations in Toronto, Ontario (Thurston et al. 1993) and for several cities in New York State (Thurston et al. 1992). The focus of these studies was the effects of acid aerosols, but estimates were reported for various measures of particle exposure. Taken together, these studies found an increase in hospital admissions for respiratory diagnoses ranging from approximately 0.8 percent to 3.4 percent for each 10 $\mu g/m^3$ increase in daily mean PM_{10}.

Several studies have also analyzed emergency department visits and found them to be associated with particulate air pollution. For example, particulate air pollution was associated with emergency department visits for asthma in Seattle, WA (Schwartz et al. 1993), emergency department visits for chronic obstructive pulmonary disease in Barcelona (Sunyer et al. 1991, 1993), and emergency department visits in Steubenville, OH (Samet et al. 1981). The estimated percent increase in emergency visits associated with a 10 $\mu g/m^3$ increase in PM_{10} ranged from 0.5 percent to 3.4 percent with a weighted mean of approximately 1.0 percent. These are summarized in Table 6.2

Given the associations between particulate pollution and emergency department visits, it would be expected that associations would also be observed for outpatient visits for respiratory illness. There is less availability of outpatient data to researchers than there is for hospitalization data. However, based on a limited study of outpatient data from a clinic in Salt Lake City, UT, Lutz (1983) reported that strong positive associations were observed between weekly particulate pollution levels and the percentage of patients with a diagnosis of respiratory tract or cardiac illness.

Exacerbation of asthma

Evidence from hospital admissions and emergency visit studies suggests that exposures to particulate air pollution may be directly associated with asthma attacks. Several investigators have considered less severe asthmatic attacks as reported by panels of asthma patients. Winter studies of asthmatic children with chronic respiratory symptoms in The Netherlands (Roemer et al. 1993) and of asthmatic adults in Denver, Colorado, (Ostro et al. 1991) both found substantial increases in reported asthmatic attacks associated with particle exposures. An earlier study in the Los Angeles area (Whittemore and Korn 1980) reported increased attacks associated with particle exposures but the effect was much lower than in the more recent studies. In part this lower effect estimate may reflect over-control of lagged effects of particles by including the previous day's asthma status in the model. The weighted mean of these three studies, however, gives an effect estimate of 3 percent increase in asthmatic attacks associated with 10 $\mu g/m^3$ increase in PM_{10} (see Table 6.3).

Bronchodilator use has also been evaluated as a measure of exacerbation of asthma in a panel of asthmatics in the Netherlands (Roemer et al. 1993) and in the Utah Valley (Pope et al. 1991). Based on the reported results of these studies, the estimated percent increase in asthma attacks or use of bronchodilator associated with a 10 $\mu g/m^3$ increase in PM_{10}

TABLE   6.3

Summary of Acute Effect of Particles on Exacerbation of Asthma

Response	Location	Reference	Particulate Measure	Subjects	% increase in asthma per 10$\mu g/m^3$ increase in PM_{10} (95% CI)
Bronchodilator use	Utah Valley	Pope et al. (1991)	PM_{10}	School panel Asthma panel	11.2 (2.4, 20.7) 12.0 (4.7,19.7)
	2 Dutch cities	Roemer et al. (1993)	PM_{10} (daily mean)	School panel	2.3 (0.7,3.8)
Asthmatic attacks	2 Dutch cities	Roemer et al. (1993)	PM_{10} (3-day mean)	School panel	1.1 (-3.5,5.9)
	Denver, CO	Ostro et al. (1991)	$PM_{2.5}$	Asthma Panel	11.5 (8.9,14.3)

range from 1.1 percent to 12 percent with a weighted mean of approximately 3.0 percent.

Respiratory symptoms

The use of daily diaries to record respiratory symptoms is an inexpensive method of evaluating acute changes in respiratory health status. In a commonly applied study design, panels of school children recorded the presence of specific respiratory symptoms in daily diaries. Symptom reports are often aggregated into upper respiratory symptoms (including such symptoms as runny or stuffy nose, sinusitis, sore throat, wet cough, head cold, hay fever, and burning or red eyes) and lower respiratory symptoms (including wheezing, dry cough, phlegm, shortness of breath, and chest discomfort or pain). In addition, cough, the most frequently reported symptom, is often analyzed separately.

Studies of upper and lower respiratory symptoms have been conducted in the Utah Valley (Pope et al. 1991, Pope and Dockery 1992), the Netherlands (Hoek & Brunekreef 1993, 1994), a study of six U.S. cities (Schwartz et al. 1994), and Southern California (Ostro et al. 1993). Very small, often statistically insignificant associations between particulate pollution and upper respiratory symptoms were observed. The association with lower respiratory disease was larger and usually statistically significant. Based on these studies, the estimated percent increase in reported lower respiratory symptoms associated with a 10 $\mu g/m^3$ increase in PM_{10} was as high as 15 percent, but the weighted mean was approximately 3.0 percent.

Cough was analyzed separately in three of these studies as well as in another diary study in the Netherlands (Roemer et al. 1993), a study of two Swiss cities (Braun-Fahrlander et al. 1992), and a study in Uniontown, Pennsylvania (Neas et al. 1992). Cough was typically associated with particulate pollution, with the estimated percent increase in reported cough associated with a 10 $\mu g/m^3$ increase in PM_{10} as high as 28 percent but with a weighted mean of approximately 1.2 percent.

Lung function

Several studies have observed negative associations between particulate pollution and lung function (see Table 6.4). Panels of elementary school children in Steubenville, OH had their lung function measured weekly before, during, and after four distinct episodes, (particles and SO_2) which occurred between 1978 and 1980 (Dockery et al. 1982). Declines in forced expiratory volume in 0.75 seconds ($FEV_{0.75}$) were observed following these episodes. In a re-analysis of the Steubenville data, Brunekreef et al. (1991)

T A B L E   6 . 4

Summary of Acute Effect of Particles on Reduction of Lung Function

Response	Location	Reference	Particulate Measure	% decrease in daily lung function per 10µg/m³ increase in PM$_{10}$ (95% CI)
FEV 0.75	Steubenville, OH	Dockery et al.(1982)	TSP	0.05 (0.00, 0.10)
FEV 1	4 Cities, NL	Hoek & Brunekeef (1993)	PM$_{10}$	0.06 (-0.01, 0.14)
FEV 1	Wageningen, NL	Hoek & Brunekeef (1993)	PM$_{10}$	0.35 (0.23, 0.48)
FEV 1	Salt Lake City, UT	Pope & Kanner (1993)	PM$_{10}$	0.21 (0.05, 0.37)
PEF	Utah Valley, UT	Pope et al. (1991)	PM$_{10}$	0.25 (0.10, 0.39)
PEF	Utah Valley, UT	Pope and Dockery (1992)	PM$_{10}$	0.06 (0.00, 0.12) 0.04 (-0.02, 0.09)
PEF	Wageningen, NL	Roemer et al. (1993)	PM$_{10}$	0.09 (-0.01, 0.20)
PEF	Uniontown, PA	Neas et al. (1992)	PM$_{10}$	0.19 (0.01, 0.37)
PEF	4 Cities, NL	Hoek & Brunekeef (1993)	PM$_{10}$	0.16 (0.05.0.28)
PEF	Wageningen, NL	Hoek & Brunekeef (1993)	PM$_{10}$	0.16 (-0.03, 0.36)

Source: updated from Dockery and Pope 1994.

found the strongest association with the mean particle concentrations over the previous 5 days. Similar decreases in forced expired volume in 1 second (FEV$_1$) were observed in school children following a particulate and sulfur oxide pollution episode in January 1985 in the Netherlands (Dassen et al. 1986). Subsequent studies of panels of school children in the Netherlands with weekly lung function measurements (Hoek & Brunekreef 1993, 1994) have also shown decreased FEV$_1$ associated with daily PM$_{10}$ concentrations. Lagged effects of up to seven days were observed.

Pope and Kanner (1993) analyzed repeated FEV$_1$ measurements in a panel of adults with chronic pulmonary disease who were participating in the Lung Health Study. Measurements were taken 10 to 90 days apart.

FEV_1 levels were found to be associated with PM_{10} concentrations. Koenig and colleagues (1993) studied the lung function [forced vital capacity (FVC) and FEV_1] of children in Seattle, WA with relatively low particulate air pollution levels. Lung function declines were associated with fine particulate air pollution for asthmatic children, but not for non-asthmatic children. Overall, these studies generally observed a decrease of up to 0.35 percent in FEV_1 associated with each 10 $\mu g/m^3$ increase in daily mean PM_{10}, with a weighted average of 0.15 percent.

Several studies have used peak flow measurements as an indicator of acute changes in lung function including studies in the Netherlands (Hoek and Brunekreef 1993, 1994; Roemer et al. 1993), the Utah Valley (Pope et al., 1991; Pope and Dockery 1992), and Uniontown, PA (Neas et al. 1992). In these studies a 10 $\mu g/m^3$ increase in PM_{10} was associated with a 0.04 percent to 0.25 percent decrease in peak flow measurements. As with FEV_1, the strongest associations with peak flow included particulate pollution over the previous several days, allowing for a lag in effect.

The reduction of lung function will be discussed further in Chapter 7 as a chronic effect and in Chapter 9 where a model is proposed whereby it might be an intermediate cause of mortality.

Restricted activity

Associations between particulate air pollution and more general measures of acute disease have also been observed. For example, Ostro (1983, 1987, 1990) and Ostro and Rothschild (1989) evaluated the timing of restricted activity days of U.S. adult workers. Restricted activity due to respiratory morbidity was consistently associated with particulate pollution. Morbidity was often more strongly associated with the fine, respirable, or sulfate component of particulate pollution. Ransom and Pope (1992) reported similar associations between PM_{10} and grade-school absences in children in the Utah Valley, Utah. Lagged pollution effects of up to several weeks were observed for both restricted activity in adults and in school absences.

Chinese Studies

A number of studies looking at various health endpoints in relation to air pollution have been done in Beijing, China. While the results are interesting, they are hard to compare to U.S. studies, and are therefore described in this separate section. Ambient levels of the pollutants measured are reported as having mean values of 388 $\mu g/m^3$ TSP and 119 $\mu g/m^3$ SO_2, and maximums at 1,255 $\mu g/m^3$ for TSP and 478 $\mu g/m^3$ for SO_2 (Xu et al. 1995a). Differences in disease classifications between China and the U.S. also exist, but as the authors suggest, these differences may actually lead to insights, if examined carefully. In Xu et al. 1994, significant associations between a doubling in SO_2 were found with deaths recorded as due to chronic obstructive pulmonary disease, pulmonary heart disease, and cardiovascular disease. The relationship between deaths from cancer and air pollution was not significant. A doubling in TSP was associated with significant increases in chronic obstructive pulmonary disease.

   In all of the studies there was a strong seasonal variation, which the authors suggest is related to the lack of air conditioning in Chinese buildings, which leads to a greater mixing of indoor and outdoor air in the summer when the windows are open. Smokestacks tend to be much shorter in China than in the U.S., causing higher ground level SO_2 and proportionally higher SO_2 to particle ratio in urban air pollution. The efforts to reduce SO_2 in the U.S. have been fairly successful, making the difference in ambient levels between the two countries even more marked.

   The prevalence of coal burning stoves in Chinese households is part of the reason for the large ambient TSP levels. A general survey conducted in Beijing showed that the contribution of natural dust is 40 to 60 percent of TSP (Wang 1981). If soil particles were discounted, the airborne particulate concentrations due to domestic, industrial and commercial coal would still result in ambient concentrations several times higher than the levels measured in the U.S. If fine combustion particles are the major factor in air pollution related health effects, using the combined measure of TSP values will significantly underestimate these health effects, as what people are breathing in consistent amounts in close quarters is dominated by the fine fraction. A study that surveyed 1,440 never-smoking Beijing residents found coal heating an "important risk factor for pulmonary function" as well as a "major confounding factor in the analysis of outdoor air pollution data" (Xu et al. 1991).

   Chinese studies used outpatient information since appointments in Beijing are not scheduled in advance, and people report to the closest facility; in China, hospital records "provide reliable information on morbidity for a geographically defined population." Significant associations were found with non-surgery visits, both outpatient and emergency room, and there was no evidence of influenza epidemics during the study periods.

Limitations and Concerns

   There are four major areas of concern pertaining to the inherent limitations of these epidemiologic studies of air pollution:

■ Issues related to methodologic or analytic bias

■ Issues relating to biologic significance or plausibility

■ Concerns about confounding by non-pollution factors

■ Determining the constituent(s) of air pollution responsible for effects

Methodological issues

As observed effects get smaller, methodological issues become progressively more important. They were comparatively irrelevant for the London air pollution incident shown in Figure 1.1, but for air pollution concentrations that are 30 to 50 times smaller they may explain, exaggerate or mask any effect. These methodological issues are discussed in some detail in Pope (1996a).

The studies reviewed in this chapter have typically used some form of time-series research methodology. They have tried to use appropriate statistical approaches to analyze the data. Some of the most compelling evidence of health effects of particulate air pollution required only very simple analysis—such as early studies that compared cardiopulmonary mortality before, during and after major pollution episodes. Many recent studies have tried to employ simple comparative statistical approaches to presenting the data but most have also employed increasingly advanced biostatistical and econometric modeling techniques to analyze the data. Critics have often suggested that the statistical methods and study designs were inadequate (Moolgavkar and Luebeck 1996). However, continued research and calculations with increasingly sophisticated methods have yielded almost the identical results. The most commonly used modeling technique that has been used is multivariate regression modeling. There are at least two primary reasons that multivariate regression models are so useful to analyze epidemiological data on the health effects of air pollution: 1) they allow for the estimation of the health-particulate associations while controlling for at least some other risk factors, and 2) they can, when used appropriately, add additional rigor to the analysis by providing a way to conduct formal hypothesis testing and more formally make statistical inferences. A detailed discussion of these analytic techniques for time-series is given by Pope and Schwartz (1996).

Because individual studies necessarily have methodological restrictions, judgements concerning the validity of these studies must involve evaluating the body of research as a whole. Various reviews have concluded that the consistency of findings from many differing study designs, data sets, and analytic techniques make it unlikely that the overall particulate air pollution effects observed could be due to systematic methodologic or analytic bias (US EPA 1996, Dockery and Pope 1994, Schwartz 1994e, Ostro 1993, Pope et al. 1995a, 1995b, Lipfert 1994).

Biologic plausibility

The results of epidemiologic studies of acute effects of particulate air pollution, particularly those describing associations with cardiovascular mortality, have been called into question because of the lack of understanding of biological mechanisms (Utell 1993, Waller 1992). Many authors have suggested that air pollution episodes, like episodes of extreme temperature, high or low, are an additional environmental stress that may cause death in otherwise compromised patients. Bates (1992) has suggested three additional explanations by which respiratory and cardiovascular mortality might increase in air pollution episodes: (a) acute bronchitis and bronchiolitis may be misdiagnosed as pulmonary edema; (b) air pollutants may increase lung permeability and precipitate pulmonary edema in people with myocardial damage and increased left atrial pressure; (c) bronchiolitis or pneumonia induced by air pollution, in the presence of preexisting heart disease, might precipitate congestive heart failure. Seaton et al. (1995) recently suggested that air pollution, specifically ultra-fine particles may provoke alveolar inflammation which, with the release of mediators, may exacerbate lung disease and increase blood coagulability. Such mechanisms may, at least in part, explain the increase in cardiovascular deaths associated with particulate air pollution.

It has also been suggested that respiratory causes of death, either primary or contributing, are reported as cardiovascular. In a summary of a workshop of chronic obstructive pulmonary disease mortality, Speizer (1989) observed that chronic obstructive pulmonary disease is considerably under diagnosed on death certificates. While the specific biologic mechanism for these acute increases in mortality is not clear and remains unconfirmed, Hill (1965) argued that it cannot always be demanded. But Hill does suggest that consistency is important. There *is* internal consistency of the mortality studies and the external consistency with evidence of acute increases in mortality measures. Biological plausibility is enhanced by the observation of a coherent cascade of cardiopulmonary health effects in epidemiologic studies, and by the fact that non-cardiopulmonary health effects are not typically associated with particulate pollution. This is discussed further in Chapters 8 and 10.

Confounding by non-pollution factors

A basic limitation of the epidemiological studies involves the difficulty of disentangling independent effects or potential interactions between highly correlated risk factors. The difficulty of disentangling independent effects or interactions exists largely because alternative risk factors may be correlated with air pollution resulting in potential confounding. Confounding may result when another risk factor that is correlated with both exposure and disease is not adequately controlled for in the analysis, resulting in spurious correlations. Although any single epidemiology study is highly limited in its ability to deal with all potential confounders, the broader body of epidemiological evidence provides some important information.

Cigarette smoking, for example, contributes to baseline or underlying respiratory disease rates in a population, but it is not likely serving as a common confounder across the epidemiologic studies of PM_{10} air pollution. Cigarette smoking would not be a confounder in the acute exposure studies for several reasons: 1) Most of the lung function, respiratory symptoms, and school absences studies were conducted among non-smoking children. 2) The largest association between respiratory hospitalizations and pollution was often with non-smoking children. 3) Cigarette smoking does not change day-to-day, week-to-week, or month-to-month in positive correlation with air pollution. As with cigarette smoking, socioeconomic status in a population does not change day-to-day in correlation with air pollution. Therefore, socioeconomic variables are not likely confounders in the short-term time-series studies looking at lung function, respiratory symptoms, school absences, outpatient visits, and mortality.

In the acute exposure studies, confounding due to temporal correlations between pollution, weather, and seasonal variables is a concern. However, independent pollution effects are typically observed even after using various approaches to control for weather variables in the regression model. For example, it has been suggested that these acute exposure studies have been compromised because they did not use synoptic weather modeling to control for weather in the regression models. However, two recent analyses of effects of air pollution on daily mortality explored the use of synoptic weather modeling (Pope and Kalkstein 1996, and Samet et al. 1996). The use of this weather modeling approach did not substantively change the estimated mortality effects of air pollution. Furthermore, estimated pollution effects are reasonably consistent for areas with very different climates and weather conditions.

Responsible constituent(s)

Another concern related to these studies is the difficulty of fully exploring the relative health impacts of various constituents of air pollution. Various measures or estimates of particulate pollution mass, for example, may only be serving in proxy for a primary toxic component or characteristic of air pollution. As presented in Chapter 5, animal and controlled human studies have suggested for many years that combustion-source fine particles, including sulfates, nitrates, some particulate acidity and metals, likely play a role. The independent effect of various air pollutants continues to be studied. Two basic approaches to evaluating the independent effect of a given pollutant can be used. One approach is to try to analytically control for co-pollutants by including them in regression models and using statistical criteria such as significance levels or coefficient size and stability to evaluate independent impact. Dockery and Schwartz, analyzed a subset of the daily mortality studies and the results are presented in Table 5.5 In this table, the coefficient relating mortality to PM_{10} was calculated in two ways: 1) by assuming that PM_{10} alone was responsible (including only PM_{10} in the regression model), and 2) by assuming that either SO_2, CO, or O_3 were co-pollutants (including the co-pollutants into the regression model). The overall coefficient is slightly reduced but still positive and statistically significant.

Moolgavkar et al. (1995) reanalyzed the Steubenville data, and also provided to Samet, Zeger and Berhane (1995) a larger data set for Philadelphia than that previously analyzed. Samet et al. find that there is an apparent correlation with SO_2 concentrations as well as with TSP correlations. The suggestion they make is that SO_2 itself may be a responsible constituent for a part of the mortality. Alternatively, SO_2 may be a surrogate for the finer fraction of TSP.

There are often strong correlations between the various pollutants making analytic control techniques replete with statistical problems. Attempts to separate effects of a single pollutant are rarely conclusive for any single data set. Fortunately, with respect to particulate pollution across various study areas, there is substantial variability in the levels of co-pollutants and the degree of co-linearity of these co-pollutants with PM. Therefore, a second and more compelling approach is to compare the estimated PM effects in areas with different potential for confounding or interaction by co-pollutants. If the estimated PM effects are due to confounding by co-pollutants, then estimated PM effects would be larger in areas with higher potential for positive confounding by co-pollutants. Analyses of this type have been conducted that provide evidence the

TABLE 6.5

Summary of Daily Time Series Studies When Considered Alone (Univariate Analysis) and with Control (Joint Analysis) of Specific Pollutants

Location	Reference	Percent increase in mortality per $10\mu g/m^3$ increase in PM_{10} (95% CI)	
		Univariate	Joint
Co-pollutant: SO₂			
Philadelphia,PA	Schwartz & Dockery (1992a)	1.2 (0.7, 1.7)	0.9 (0.3, 1.6)
Detroit, MI	Schwartz (1991)	1.0 (0.5, 1.6)	0.9 (0.4,1.5)
Steubenville,OH	Schwartz & Dockery (1992b)	0.6 (0.2, 1.0)	0.5 (0.1, 1.0)
Athens, Greece	Toulomi et al. (1994)	0.9 (0.7, 1.2)	0.5 (0.1, 1.9)
Erfut, Germany	Spix et al. (1994)	0.6 (0.1, 1.1)	0.5 (-0.1, 1.1)
Sao Paulo, Braz.	Saldiva et al. (1995)	1.3 (0.7, 1.9)	1.4 (0.4, 2.5)
Amsterdam, ND	Verhoeff et al. (1996)	0.6 (-0.1, 1.4)	0.2 (-0.8, 1.2)
Combined		0.9 (0.7, 1.0)	0.7 (0.5, 0.9)
Co-pollutant: CO			
Athens, Greece	Toulomi et al. (1994)	0.9 (0.7, 1.2)	0.8 (0.4, 1.2)
Los Angeles, USA	Kinney et al. (1995)	0.5 (0.0, 1.0)	0.4 (-0.1, 0.9)
Amsterdam, ND	Verhoeff et al. (1996)	0.6 (-0.1, 1.4)	1.0 (0.1, 1.9)
Combined		0.8 (0.6,1.0)	0.7 (0.4,1.0)
Co-pollutant: O₃			
Sao Paulo, Braz.	Saldiva et al. (1995)	1.3 (0.7, 1.9)	1.4 (0.4, 2.5)
Los Angeles, USA	Kinney et al. (1995)	0.5 (0.0, 1.0)	0.5 (0.0, 1.0)
Amsterdam, ND	Verhoeff et al. (1996)	0.6 (-0.1, 1.4)	0.3 (-0.6, 1.2)
Combined		0.8 (0.4, 1.1)	0.6 (0.2, 1.0)

Source: Dockery and Schwartz 1996.

observed PM effects are largely independent of O_3, or SO_2. (Schwartz 1996, Pope 1996b).

With respect to particulate air pollution, various physiologic and toxicologic concerns suggest that particulate pollution from combustion sources (including sulfate and nitrate particles) may be a larger health concern than naturally occurring particles (see Chapter 5). Their size is such that they can be breathed most deeply in the lungs and they include sulfates, nitrates, acids, transitional metals, and carbon particles with various chemicals adsorbed onto their surfaces. Also, relative to coarse particles, indoor and personal exposure to combustion-source fine particles are much better represented by central site ambient monitors. Long-term transport and large-scale mixing of combustion products result in concentrations of combustion related particles that are relatively uniform within communities (see Chapters 2 and 3). Penetration of fine combustion-source particles also results in measured indoor and personal exposures to sulfate and fine particles being strongly correlated with and similar to measured outdoor concentrations (see Chapter 4).

Much of the epidemiological evidence is consistent with the expectation that combustion-source air pollution may be a larger health risk than naturally occurring particles. The increased mortality and morbidity associated with early severe episode studies in Donora, Muese Valley, and London occurred during stagnant air conditions (Firket 1931, Ciocco and Thompson 1961, Logan 1953). The PM pollution was primarily combustion-source particles (often simply referred to as smoke). Because of the strong temporal correlation between measures of fine, respirable, sulfate, or total suspended particles in many study areas, daily time-series studies often have a difficult time separating out effects of fine versus course particles. For example, in the daily time-series mortality analysis of St. Louis and Eastern Tennessee (Dockery et al. 1992), mortality was not strongly associated with aerosol acidity, O_3, NO_2, or SO_2; however, mortality was associated with but both fine and course particles. Schwartz et al. (1996) conducted a daily time-series mortality study using mortality and air pollution data from six U.S. cities. They observed that, in general, mortality was much more strongly associated with $PM_{2.5}$ compared to course particles (PM_{15}–$PM_{2.5}$), sulfate particles, or acid aerosols. Other time-series studies have observed that combustion-source particles are more strongly associated with health endpoints. For example, another daily time-series study reported that respiratory hospital admissions in Toronto were more strongly associated with combustion related particles such as fine, sulfate, and acidic particles (Thurston et al. 1993).

A common feature of time-series studies of mortality in urban areas is that a large component of the particulate pollution is produced either directly or indirectly in combustion processes. There are few comparable time-series studies of naturally occurring crustal or soil derived particles that are not part of a complex pollution mix that includes combustion particles. A study in southeast Washington State evaluated emergency room visits for respiratory illness associated with very high daily PM_{10} concentrations (>1000 $\mu g/m^3$) due to wind-blown dust (Hefflin et al. 1994). Relatively small associations with bronchitis and sinusitis were observed and visits for total respiratory disorders were not associated with particle levels. Another study evaluated the pulmonary function of school children after exposure to high levels of volcanic ash (Johnson et al. 1990). TSP during the highest 24-hour period exceeded 10,000 $\mu g/m^3$ and fine particle concentrations (≤ 2.5 μm) for the same 24-hour period equaled 112 $\mu g/m^3$. No substantial decrease in pulmonary function was observed associated with the volcanic ash episode. However, significant declines in lung function were observed after 3 days exposure to urban particulate pollution at much smaller concentrations (3-day average TSP equaled 440 $\mu g/m^3$).

Role of particulate acidity

Chapter 5 discusses the animal evidence that indicates an important role of combustion metals, sulfur oxides in combination with other pollutants. Several of the time series studies have observed health effects associated with sulfates and in Chapter 7 it will be noted that increased mortality has been associated with chronic exposure to fine particulate air pollution including sulfates. Spengler et al. (1990) and EPA (1989) review the evidence supporting the involvement of particle sulfur acidity. But the current view is more complicated than can be explained by a single pollutant entity. Although sulfate levels may be viewed as "potential acidity," in many areas with substantial levels of sulfates, there may be very low acidity due to neutralization by alkaline coals, ammonia and the production of neutral salt species (Brauer et al. 1995). Therefore, sulfate concentrations may not necessarily be a better proxy for levels of aerosol acidity than it is for combustion-source fine particles more generally defined. Furthermore, while sulfate particles penetrate indoors (Dockery and Spengler 1981, Suh et al. 1992) substantial neutralization in indoor environments results in lower actual exposures to acidity than what would be inferred from outdoor and a simple penetration factor P (Brauer et al. 1991).

The epidemiological evidence seems to suggest that the health-particulate relationship may be largely independent of acidity. Time-series studies that have been conducted with the objective to evaluate the role of acid aerosols, fine particles, or sulfate particles typically have made one of three observations: 1) there is remarkably little measurable aerosol acidity, but adverse health effects are often associated with measures of inhalable, fine, or sulfate particles anyway (Pope et al. 1991, Brauer et al. 1995); 2) aerosol acidity is present, but it is not as strongly associated with adverse health effects as other proxy measures of combustion-source particles (Dockery et al. 1992, Schwartz et al. 1996); 3) aerosol acidity is present, but it is strongly correlated with fine particles and sulfate particles and all of these measures are associated with the health endpoints (Thurston et al. 1993, Ostro et al. 1991). Furthermore, the estimated associations between fine particles and adverse health effects are not generally higher in areas with relative high levels of aerosol acidity versus areas with low levels of aerosol acidity.

The contrast between the apparent importance of acidity suggested in Chapter 5 and the lack of epidemiological evidence therefore is an important issue for future study.

Summary

Evidence from the selected epidemiologic studies presented in this review suggests a coherence of effects across a range of related health outcomes and a consistency of effects across independent studies with different investigators in different settings. This compilation also provides insights into the relative magnitude of effects being observed in various studies.

Total mortality is observed to increase by approximately 1 percent per 10 $\mu g/m^3$ increase in PM_{10}. Somewhat stronger associations are observed for cardiovascular mortality (approximately 1.4 percent per 10 $\mu g/m^3$ PM_{10}) and considerably stronger associations are observed for respiratory mortality (approximately 3.4 percent per 10 $\mu g/m^3$ PM_{10}). Acute effects with cancer and other nonpulmonary and noncardiovascular causes of mortality were not consistently observed.

If respiratory mortality is associated with particulate pollution, then health care visits for respiratory illness would also be expected to be associated with particulate pollution. Respiratory hospital admissions and emergency department visits increase by approximately 0.8 percent and 1.0 percent per 10 $\mu g/m^3$ PM_{10} respectively. Emergency department visits for asthmatics (3.4 percent increase per 10 $\mu g/m^3$ PM_{10}) and hospital admissions for asthmatic attacks (1.9 percent increase per 10 $\mu g/m^3$ PM_{10}) are more strongly associated. Asthmatic subjects also report substantial increases in asthma attacks (an approximate 3 percent increase per 10 $\mu g/m^3$ PM_{10}) and in bronchodilator use (an approximate 3 percent increase per 10 $\mu g/m^3$ PM_{10}).

Less severe measures of respiratory health also are associated with particle exposures. Lower respiratory symptom reporting increases by approximately 3.0 percent per 10 $\mu g/m^3$ PM_{10} and cough by 2.5 percent per 10 $\mu g/m^3$ PM_{10}. Weaker effects are observed with upper respiratory symptoms (approximately 0.7 percent per 10 $\mu g/m^3$ PM_{10}). While lung function provides accurate objective measures, the observed mean effects are fairly modest: approximately 0.15 percent decrease for FEV_1 or $FEV_{0.75}$ and 0.08 percent decrease for peak flow per 10 µg/m³ PM_{10}. Despite the relatively small size of these lung-function effect estimates, they are often statistically significance. Moreover, mean changes in lung function may not reflect substantial changes in sensitive individuals.

In this review, changes in health measures are reported even for small changes in daily particulate pollution: 10 µg/m³ increase in PM_{10} concentrations. Because daily concentrations of PM_{10} in some US cities average over 50 µg/m³ and often exceed 100 or 150 µg/m³, the effects of particulate pollution can be substantial for realistic acute exposures. For example, a coefficient of 1 percent effect per each 10 µg/m³ increase would produce a 5 percent increase in the health measure for a 50 µg/m³ increase in PM_{10} concentrations (which increase is not uncommon), and a coefficient of 3 percent per 10 µg/m³ PM_{10}, which is the estimated coefficient for asthma attacks would lead to a 16 percent increase in asthma attacks for a 50 µg/m³ increase in PM_{10} concentrations.

The epidemiological studies of the health effects of acute exposures to air pollution have both strengths and limitations that stem largely from the use of people who are living in uncontrolled environments, and who are exposed to complex mixtures of air pollution. The pattern of cardio-pulmonary health outcomes associated with acute exposure to air pollution that has come from these epidemiological studies is one important set of evidence. A more complete understanding of the acute health effects of particulate air pollution will require important contributions from toxicology, exposure assessment, and other disciplines. Nevertheless, the epidemiological studies of acute exposure to air pollution provide substantial evidence that combustion-related air pollution may be a risk factor for pulmonary disease and can exacerbate existing cardiovascular and pulmonary disease and increase the number of persons in a population who become symptomatic, require medical attention, or die.

7

Epidemiology of Chronic Health Effects: Cross-Sectional Studies

Arden Pope and Douglas Dockery

Introduction

In Chapter 6 we discussed the acute effects of air pollution on mortality and morbidity. These are the effects that are associated with short-term (often day-to-day) changes in levels of air pollution. In this chapter we discuss the effects of chronic or long-term exposure to air pollution. Chronic effects may include effects of low or moderate exposure that persists for a long time as well as the cumulative effects of repeated exposure to elevated levels of pollution. Small effects of acute exposure might accumulate over longer periods of time to produce a major chronic effect upon health. The existence of an acute effect of air pollution does not automatically imply that there is a chronic effect and vice-versa. However, the existence of one, may make the existence of the other more plausible.

Available chronic exposure studies compare mortality and morbidity health outcomes among communities with different levels of air pollution. These studies use longer-term pollution data (usually 1 year or more). Because of the extended time period and the geographical cross-sectional design of these studies, they are typically interpreted as evaluating chronic or cumulative effects of exposure. The health effects observed in these studies may include cumulative acute effects discussed in Chapter 6 (provided that the acute effects persist down to normal ambient levels), in addition to chronic effects such as cancer or chronic cardiopulmonary disease which have long latent periods and would not show up in time series studies. As noted before in Figure 6.1, the chronic exposure studies include population-based studies and cohort studies and look at various health outcomes. Recent cross-sectional studies of air pollution have also reported associations between particulate pollution and respiratory symptoms, lung function, and mortality rates (Table 7.1).

T A B L E   7 . 1

Summary of Selected Chronic Mortality and Morbidity Studies

Health Indicator	Study Design	Reference	Brief Summary of Findings
Mortality Rates	Population-based cross-sectional mortality studies	Lave, Seskin 1970 Chappie, Lave 1982 Lipfert 1984 Evans et al. 1984 Ozkaynak, Thurston 1987 Lipfert et al. 1988 Archer 1990 Bobak, Leon 1992	Average mortality effect estimated at 3–9 percent of total U.S. mortality. Magnitude of effect sensitive to model specification, choice of social, demographic, and other variables included in the models, and the choice of study areas used in the analysis.
Lung Function	Analysis of community ambient air pollution data with individual health and risk data from national surveys or cohorts	Dockery et al. 1989 Schwartz 1989 Chestnut et al. 1991 Raizenne et al. 1993	Small, but generally statistically significant, negative associations. 10 $\mu g/m^3$ increase in PM_{10} surveys or cohorts associated with less than a 2 percent decline in lung function.
Respiratory Symptoms	Analysis of community ambient air pollution data with individual health and risk data from national surveys or collected cohorts	Euler et al. 1987 Dockery et al. 1989 Portney & Mullahy 1990 Schwartz 1993 Dockery et al. 1993	Chronic cough, bronchitis and chest illness (but not asthma) were associated with various measures of particulate air pollution. A 10 $\mu g/m^3$ increase in PM_{10} was typically associated with a10 to 25 percent increase in bronchitis or chronic cough.
Mortality (survival times)	Prospective cohort mortality studies that linked community-based air pollution data with individual risk factor and survival data	Dockery et al. 1993a Pope et al. 1995c	After controlling for individual differences in age, sex, cigarette smoking, and other risk factors, fine and/or sulfate particulate pollution was associated with mortality (mostly cardiopulmonary mortality).

Adapted from Pope, Dockery and Schwartz 1995.

Mortality Studies

Population-based (ecologic) mortality studies

There have been many studies that have suggested mortality effects of chronic exposure to air pollution. In an early study, Martin (1964) reported that in the Greater London region overall annual respiratory mortality (as opposed to episodic mortality) was significantly related to smoke (or particulate pollution) levels. In 1970 Lave and Seskin reported the results of one of the first serious attempts to measure long-term mortality effects of air pollution in the U.S.

The work of Lave and Seskin has been followed by many other similar studies that have tried to replicate or refine their use of population-based (ecologic) cross-sectional study designs. A summary of these studies is presented in Table 7.2. Most of these studies observed that on average, mortality rates tended to be higher in cities with higher fine or sulfate particulate pollution levels than in those with lower levels. Formal regression modeling techniques to evaluate cross-sectional differences in air pollution and mortality and to control for other ecological variables were used. In an attempt to control for other risk factors, population average values for demographic variables and other factors such as smoking rates, education levels, income levels, poverty rates, housing density, and others were often included in the regression models. The basic conclusions from the population-based cross-sectional studies include:

■ Mortality rates are associated with air pollution.

■ Mortality rates are most strongly associated with fine or sulfate particulate matter.

■ An average mortality effect of 3 to 9 percent of total mortality can be estimated.

■ Typically, coefficients of air pollution–related mortality of about 3 per cent per 10 μg/m^3 were derived.

Limitations of population-based studies

Although these population-based cross-sectional studies suggest that air pollution contributes to human mortality, these studies have severe limitations and have been largely discounted for several reasons. An overriding concern of these studies was their "ecological" design and the potential for "ecological bias" as mentioned in the introduction and discussed briefly in Chapter 6. Another reason for the hesitation in using

TABLE 7.2

Selected Population-Based Cross-Sectional Studies of Mortality Effects of Chronic Exposure to Particulate Pollution

Author/Year	Study Areas	Brief Summary of Reported Findings
Lave and Seskin 1977 Chappie & Lave 1982 Lipfert 1984 Evans et al. 1984	U.S. SMSAs	Associations between mortality and particulate pollution were observed. The relationship between mortality and particulate pollution was sensitive to model specification, choice of social, demographic, and other variables included in the models, and the choice of SMSAs used in the analysis.
Özkaynak & Thurston 1987	U.S. SMSAs	Associations between mortality and particulate concentrations were and consistent with sulfate and fine particles. Particles from iron/steel industry and coal combustion larger contributors to human mortality than soil derived particles.
Mendelsohn & Orcutt 1979	U.S. County groups	Associations between mortality and sulfate particulates. Smaller, less consistent associations with CO and SO_2. An estimated 9% of total mortality was associated with air pollution.
Lipfert et al. 1988	U.S. Cities	SO_4, SO_2, NO_x, fine particles, and particulate trace metals (FE and Mn) associated with mortality. Effects of SO_4, fine particles fairly consistent.
Archer 1990	Three counties in Utah	Spatial and longitudinal differences in death rates in three counties with low smoking rates and the introduction of a major pollution source were evaluated. It was estimated that 30–40% of respiratory disease deaths (approximately 5% of all deaths) were associated with the air pollution in the most polluted county.
Bobak & Lean 1992	Czech Republic Districts	Infant mortality associated with particulate air pollution (PM_{10}). Adjusting for socioeconomic characteristics, relative risk of respiratory post-neonatal mortality was approximately 3.00 for most polluted areas versus least polluted areas.

Adapted from Pope, Bates, and Raizenne 1995.

these studies as definitive is the size of the estimated association. If taken literally, these studies suggested that as much as 3 to 9% of urban mortality in the U.S. is associated with contemporary particulate air pollution. Since air pollution in the U.S. is now relatively low, compared with air pollution in cities in previous centuries, such a large mortality effect would seem, at first sight, to imply an extraordinary effect in previous centuries and therefore implausible. Much of the chronic exposure to the elderly people now dying occurred in earlier years when concentrations were much higher, and the mortality effects applicable to current pollutant levels may be overestimated, therefore, the study design and models that predict such a large effect must be tested and retested. Confidence in the results of the population-based (ecologic) mortality studies was also limited because the strength of the estimated pollution effect was sensitive to model specification, the choice of social, demographic, and other variables included in the models, and the choice of study areas used in the analysis.

A more explicit limitation of the cross-sectional population-based studies is a prevailing concern that the observed association was due to confounding, or misidentification of the actual causal agent because it follows similar patterns as the measured parameter. Because of their ecologic design, these population-based cross-sectional studies could not directly control for individual differences in cigarette smoking and other risk factors. They could only try to control for them by using population-based averages—making potential confounding a concern. Confounding can be a more serious problem for the chronic health effect studies than for the acute health effect studies. To confound acute effects time-series studies, unknown causal variables would have to be correlated with pollution episodes in a similar way across several different locations. This is not very likely. On the other hand, for chronic effects cross-sectional studies, it is recognized that many health-related factors (age, poverty, health care, occupations, cigarette smoking, housing quality, cooking fuels) vary among cities and potentially could be confounding the apparent air pollution associations.

The issue of confounding is made more complex if one addresses the possibility that several causes may be synergistic in causing adverse health effects. For example, cigarette smoking is known to have major effects on health and major effects on the lung function. If fine particles act on the lung in the same way, they might add to the effect of cigarette smoking, or even multiply the effect of cigarette smoking. Some studies of the relationship between cigarette smoking and lung cancer showed larger effects in cities (which presumably had larger air pollution) than in the countryside (Stocks 1966). Inversely, different coefficients relating air pollution to health might be expected for smokers and non smokers. It has been suggested, for example, that air pollution levels might be below a "threshold" for nonsmokers, but that the pollution of cigarette smoking already brought smokers above that threshold, leading to an "incremental" effect with air pollution (Crawford and Wilson 1996), whereas there might be no effect or a smaller effect for nonsmokers. Unfortunately the distinction between smokers and non smokers is not routinely made in population statistics, and it becomes impossible to ask this question in the population-based studies.

Research needs for improved study designs

With respect to potential mortality effects of chronic exposure to air pollution, two important issues were being debated during the 1970s and 1980s. First, there was the idea of a threshold, a level of pollution below which there were no discernible health effects. Second there was the question of study design, and what sort of evidence was necessary or reliable to prove that air pollution was indeed causing health problems.

The idea of a threshold is one that arose in reaction to the extreme pollution events earlier in the century and has appeal based on its legislatability. If there is a threshold, then there is a clear level to aim for with respect to National Ambient Air Quality Standards. Without a threshold, it becomes much more difficult to establish a generally accepted goal for pollution control and mediation of effects. Thus, it is not simply a scientific question, but one that has clear repercussions and biases attached.

In an influential 1979 review of the data published between 1968 and 1977, several prominent British scientists systematically discounted the evidence presented in the ecologic studies (Holland et al. 1979). They concluded that the health effects of particulate pollution at low concentrations could not be "disentangled" from health effects of other factors. The 1982 EPA report which expounded the reasons for the change to a PM_{10} standard also dismissed these data for similar reasons, stating "the relationship between long-term exposure to air pollution has been extensively studied, but few of the studies provide sound or consistent findings sufficient to make quantitative conclusions." In the appendix to the 1982 EPA staff document on particulate matter the population studies are described as dealing with "unknown levels of exposure of ill-defined groups of individuals to unspecified pollutants for unstated periods of time, [which] fail to control for many variables known to affect health status."

Other reviewers in the 1970s and 1980s, however, contended that the cumulative weight of evidence did provide at least some evidence that human health could be adversely affected by particulate pollution, even at relatively low concentrations (Shy 1979, Bates 1980, Ellison and Waller 1978, Ware et al. 1981). Whether increased mortality is truly associated with chronic exposure to low levels of air pollution or whether there is a safe threshold where no health effects can be observed can only be answered satisfactorily by working on the second question—developing better study techniques and designs.

Prospective Cohort Mortality Studies

Recently the results of three prospective cohort mortality studies have been reported. Because of their improved study design these studies brought some of the most compelling evidence about mortality effects of chronic exposure to air pollution. Table 7.3 compares some of the major study design characteristics of the population-based and recent cohort-based mortality and chronic exposure studies. Direct observations of individual information on smoking, sex, age, occupation, and, in one study, pulmonary function have made these studies a new class of cross-sectional study. The previous studies had been population (ecologic) studies, which relied on data available for the population as a whole, such as census reports, rather than tracking the effects on specific individuals. Cohort studies analyze the incidence of health effects in a sample of individuals whose relevant personal characteristics are recorded along with the variables in question.

The two principle negative aspects of the prospective cohort studies of mortality are that they must also rely on community-based air pollution monitoring to estimate exposures to pollution and they are costly and time-consuming. They involve collecting large amounts of information on large numbers of people and following them prospectively for long

TABLE 7.3

Design Comparisons of the Population-Based and Recent Cohort-Based Mortality and Chronic Exposure Studies

Design Characteristics	Population-Based	Cohort-Based
Study Unit	Ill-defined populations of selected urban areas	Individuals enrolled in well-defined cohorts in selected communities
Health outcome data	Retrospectively collected mortality rates	Prospectively collected individual mortality data (including survival times and cause of death)
Estimates of pollution exposure	Rely on community based pollution monitoring	Rely on community based pollution monitoring
Data on alternative risk factors	Population average age, smoking rate, etc.	Individual information on age, sex, race, smoking history, BMI, occupation, etc.
Data analytic techniques	Standard cross-sectional regression analysis	Survival analysis including Cox Proportional Hazard Regression

periods of time. One recently reported prospective cohort-based mortality study is the California Seventh-Day Adventists study (Abbey et al. 1991). This study prospectively followed about 6,000 white, nonsmoking, long-term California residents for 6 to 10 years. Mortality relative to long-term cumulative exposure to total suspended particulates (TSP) and ozone was evaluated. Mortality was not consistently associated with TSP. Unfortunately this study did not have measures for respirable particulate pollution (PM_{10}) or fine particles ($PM_{2.5}$). Consequently, there are only two large prospective cohort studies that evaluate mortality effects of respirable or fine particulate air pollution in U.S. urban areas.

Harvard six-cities study

The first of these recently reported prospective-cohort mortality studies was the "Six Cities study" (Dockery et al. 1993a). This study involved a 14–16 year prospective follow-up of 8,111 adults living in 6 U.S. cities: Harriman, Tennessee; St. Louis, Missouri; Steubenville, Ohio; Portage, Wisconsin; and Topeka, Kansas. The six cities were selected to be representative of the range of particulate air pollution in the U.S. and approximately 1,400 people per city were included. Total suspended particulates (TSP), PM_{10}, $PM_{2.5}$, SO_4, H^+, SO_2, NO_2, and O_3 levels were monitored. The data were then analyzed using survival analysis, including multivariate Cox proportional hazards regression modeling. Although TSP concentrations dropped over the study periods, fine particulate and sulfate pollution concentrations were relatively constant. The most polluted city was Steubenville; the least polluted cities were Topeka and Portage. Differences in the probability of survival among the cities were statistically significant ($P < 0.01$). The Cox proportional hazards model was used to estimate adjusted mortality-rate ratios.

Mortality risks were most strongly associated with cigarette smoking, but after controlling for individual differences in age, sex, cigarette smoking, body mass index, education, and occupational exposure, differences in relative mortality risks across the six cities were strongly associated with difference in pollution levels in those cities. Associations between mortality risk and air pollution were stronger for respirable particles and sulfates, as measured by PM_{10}, $PM_{2.5}$, and SO_4, than for TSP, SO_2, acidity (H^+), or ozone. As shown in Figure 7.1 the association between mortality risk and fine particulate air pollution was consistent and nearly linear, with no apparent "no effects" threshold level above the ambient level in the least polluted city (Portage). The adjusted total mortality-rate ratio for the most polluted of the cities compared with the least polluted was

FIGURE 7.1

Estimated Adjusted Mortality Rate-Ratios from the Six-Cities Study Plotted against Non-Inhalable Particles (TSP-IP), the Coarse Fraction of Inhalable Particles (IP-FP), Fine Particles (PM$_{2.5}$), and Sulfate Particles

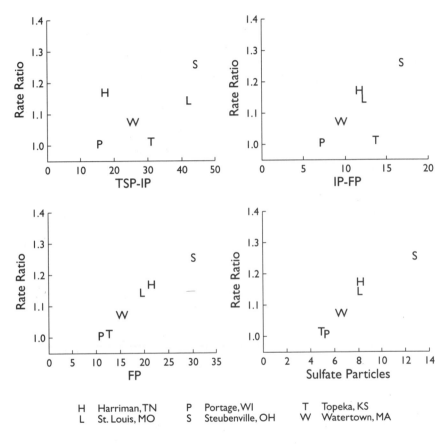

H   Harriman, TN   P   Portage, WI   T   Topeka, KS
L   St. Louis, MO   S   Steubenville, OH W   Watertown, MA

Units are μg/m³.

1.26 with 95% confidence interval (CI) from 1.08 to 1.47. Fine particulate pollution was associated with cardiopulmonary mortality and lung cancer mortality (not statistically significant) but not with the mortality due to other causes analyzed as a group.

ACS 151-city study

Similar results were observed in a much larger prospective cohort study (Pope et al. 1995c). In this study approximately 500,000 adults drawn from the American Cancer Society (ACS) Cancer Prevention Study II (CPS-II) who lived in 151 different U.S. metropolitan areas were followed prospectively from 1982 through 1989. Individual risk-factor data and 8 year vital status data were collected. Ambient concentrations of sulfates and fine particles, which are relatively consistent indoors and outdoors (see Chapter 4) were used as indices of exposure to combustion source ambient particulate air pollution. Exposure was estimated from national data bases. Pollution exposure also was assessed for a time period just prior to entry into the cohort. Both fine and sulfate particles are used as indices of combustion source particulate pollution. Adjusted mortality relative risk ratios were estimated using multiple regression analysis based on the Cox proportional hazards model. Adjusted risk ratios were calculated and reported for a difference in air pollution equal to the range of pollution exposure that existed across the metropolitan areas. Sulfate and fine particulate air pollution were associated with a difference of approximately 15 to 17 percent between total mortality risks in the most polluted cities and those in the least polluted cities.

An association between mortality and air pollution was observed after adjusting for age, sex, race, cigarette smoking, pipe and cigar smoking, exposure to passive cigarette smoke, occupational exposure, education, body mass index, and alcohol use. Additionally, weather variables that accounted for relatively hot or cold conditions were added. Adjusted mortality-rate ratios (and 95 percent confidence intervals) of total mortality for the most polluted areas compared with the least polluted equaled 1.15 (1.09–1.22) and 1.17 (1.09–1.26) when using sulfate and fine particulate measures, respectively. For total, cardiopulmonary, and lung cancer mortality, the associations with sulfate particles were highly statistically significant (P<0.01). For total and cardiopulmonary mortality, significant associations were also found using fine particulate matter as the index of air pollution levels. The association between air pollution and all-cause and cardiopulmonary mortality was observed for both men and women and for smokers and nonsmokers.

This study also compared the observed mortality rates for the cohort to U.S. area mortality rates for 1980 (NCHS 1985). This ecologic comparison, which adjusted for age, sex, and race based on 1980 census data found similar associations to those found by the prospective cohort in the same communities (U.S. Census 1983). Like the six cities study, this study included both individual data and a wider geographical area than previously possible. Geography is an important consideration that is hard to account for in models, but the development of individual histories in studies will help it be better understood. The migration of more pollution sensitive and economically mobile to lower pollution areas would cause the effects of pollution to be underestimated by population studies. The deaths of such people would be recorded in low pollution areas after they had been exposed in other places. The length of time monitored in the study may only be a proxy for the relevant chronic exposure length. It will be a good proxy if annual average fine particulate concentrations have been relatively constant or if the relevant window of exposure is only recent exposure.

Implications of prospective cohort mortality results

Previous population-based mortality studies suggested an association between mortality and sulfate and/or fine particulate air pollution. These recent prospective cohort studies confirm that these associations persist even when individual differences in age, sex, race, smoking, body mass index and other risk factors are controlled for. A summary of the results from the six-cities and ACS prospective cohort studies are presented in Table 7.4. A consistent association between mortality and cigarette smoking was observed for both studies. The increased risk associated with air pollution was small compared to that from cigarette smoking, but the evidence suggests that the association between pollution and mortality was not due to inadequate control of smoking. Even after carefully con-

TABLE 7.4

Comparisons of Mortality Risk Ratios (and 95% CI) for Smoking and Air Pollution from the 6-Cities and ACS Prospective Cohort Studies

| Cause of Death | Current Smoker* | | Particulate Air Pollution (Most- vs. Least-Polluted City) | | |
	6-Cities	ACS	6-Cities ($PM_{2.5}$)	ACS ($PM_{2.5}$)	ACS (SO_4)
All	2.00 (1.51–2.65)	2.07 (1.75–2.43)	1.26 (1.08–1.47)	1.17 (1.09–1.26)	1.15 (1.09–1.22)
Cardio-pulmonary	2.30 (1.56–3.41)	2.28 (1.79–2.91)	1.37 (1.11–1.68)	1.31 (1.17–1.46)	1.26 (1.16–1.37)
Lung Cancer	8.00 (2.97–21.6)	9.73 (5.96–15.9)	1.37 (0.81–2.31)	1.03 (0.80–1.33)	1.36 (1.11–1.66)
All others	1.46 (0.89–2.39)	1.54 (1.19–1.99)	1.01 (0.79–1.30)	1.07 (0.92–1.24)	1.01 (0.92–1.11)

* Risk ratios for current cigarette smokers with approximately 25 pack-years (about average at enrollment for both studies) compared with never-smokers.

trolling for smoking in the analysis the association with air pollution persisted. Furthermore, the association remained, even when only never smokers were included in the analysis.

The elevated mortality observed in these studies is likely to be due to both cumulative acute effects as well as chronic effects from long term exposure. If there were no chronic effect due to long term exposures and if the time series studies discussed in Chapter 6 were simply reporting deaths that would have occurred within a few day or weeks, these cross-sectional studies would not have found comparable results.

If the results from these studies are interpreted literally, the annual number of deaths in the U.S. attributed to fine particulate air pollution levels over background levels can be calculated. The actual estimates can vary substantially depending on the specific coefficients and assumptions used. For example, a recent report used the 6-cities and ACS results to estimate annual mortality attributable to fine particulate air pollution in 239 U.S. cities (NRDC 1996). The base estimate equaled approximately 64,000 deaths per year with a range of estimates between approximately 28,000 to 124,000 deaths per year. Certainly the results of these studies do not allow for air pollution related deaths to be estimated with much precision. They do, however, suggest long-term exposure to air pollution continues to be an important contributor to early mortality.

Chronic Health Effects; Morbidity

Most of the chronic epidemiological studies use death as the end-point. This is because death is a relatively objective health endpoint, whereas diagnoses of disease are more complex and subjective, with more room for bias and misclassification. Nonetheless, just as it is for the acute mortality studies, a study of morbidity health endpoints in relation to chronic exposure to air pollution is important. If particles contribute to cardiopulmonary mortality they would also likely contribute to cardiopulmonary morbidity.

Chronic differences in lung function

There is a well known reduction of lung function associated with the smoking of tobacco, and it has even been suggested that this reduction is a partial cause of subsequent morbidity and mortality. Accordingly, a search for such a reduction is an obvious necessity in any serious study of other air pollutants. Holland and Reid (1965) made a cross-sectional comparison of British male postal employees in London and in smaller country towns, where levels of SO_2 and particulate pollution were about half of those in the metropolis. Accounting for cigarette smoking levels, significant decrements of FEV_1 (Forced Expiratory Volume in 1 second) in London employees compared to those in the provinces were reported.

There have been several more recent studies that have evaluated associations between measures of lung function (Forced Vital Capacity—FVC, Forced Expiratory Volume in the first second of exhalation—FEV_1, Peak Expiratory Flow—PEF) and particulate pollution levels in the U.S. These studies include analysis of children's lung function data from the Harvard six-city study (Dockery et al. 1989), analysis of data from both the first and second National Health and Nutrition Examination Surveys (NHANES I and NHANES II) (Chestnut et al. 1991 and Schwartz 1989), and analysis of children's lung function from 24 U.S. cities (Raizenne et al. 1993). Unlike the population-based mortality studies, each of these studies had information on individual persons in the samples. The effects of air pollution on lung function were estimated after adjusting for individual differences in age, race, sex, height, and weight and controlling for smoking or restricting the analysis to never-smokers.

All of these studies observed small negative associations between lung function and particulate air pollution. In the six-cities study, which had the least statistical power, the association was very weak and statistically insignificant. In each of the other studies, the association was small, but statistically significant. The results suggest that a 10 $\mu g/m^3$ positive difference in PM_{10} was typically associated with less than a two percent decline in lung function. However, lung function measures have been shown to be important measures of health with remarkable predictive capacity for survival (Bates 1989). Furthermore, as reported in the 24-city study, the risk of relatively large deficits in lung function (15 percent or more) was much higher in the more polluted cities, suggesting detrimental effects of respirable particulates or particulate acidity on normal lung growth and development.

The possible reduction of lung function with chronic exposure to particulates is very important, because it is one of the biological mechanisms that has been proposed to account for the morbidity and mortality. This will be discussed further in Chapter 9.

Chronic respiratory symptoms and disease

There have also been several recent studies that have evaluated associations between particulate air pollution and chronic respiratory symptoms and disease. These studies include the Harvard six-cities study (Dockery et al. 1989), analysis of chronic obstructive pulmonary disease (COPD) symptoms of never-smoking Seventh-Day Adventists in California (Euler et al. 1987), analysis of data from the 1979 version of the U.S. National Health Interview Survey (NHIS) (Portney and Mullahy, 1990), analysis using data from the first National Health and Nutrition Examination Survey (NHANES I) (Schwartz 1993), and analysis of the symptoms data from the 24-cities study (Dockery et al. 1993). The effects of air pollution on respiratory disease or symptoms were estimated while adjusting for individual differences in various other risk factors.

In all of these studies, statistically significant associations were observed between particulate air pollution and respiratory symptoms. Particulate air pollution was most consistently associated with bronchitic symptoms. The results suggest that a 10 µg/m^3 increase in PM$_{10}$ was typically associated with a 10 to 25 percent increase in bronchitis or chronic cough. The results are shown in Figures 2 and 3.

FIGURE 7.2

Bronchitis in the Last Year, Children 10 to 12 Years in Age in Six U.S. Cities, by PM$_{15}$

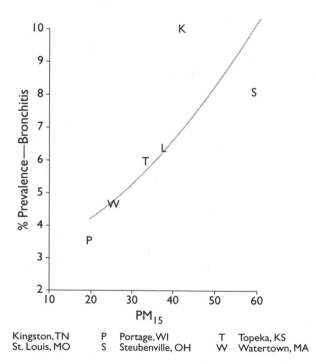

K	Kingston, TN	P	Portage, WI	T	Topeka, KS
L	St. Louis, MO	S	Steubenville, OH	W	Watertown, MA

FIGURE 7.3

Bronchitis in the Last Year, Children 10 to 12 Years in Age in Four U.S. Cities, by Hydrogen Ion Concentrations

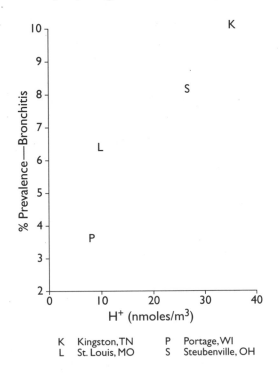

| K | Kingston, TN | P | Portage, WI |
| L | St. Louis, MO | S | Steubenville, OH |

A problem that has accompanied attempts to report long-term effects is the difficulty in determining whether the five-year average air pollution level, the twenty-five year average, or the number of peaks of a certain levels within these periods is responsible for the effects that are measured. The Seventh-Day Adventists study was followed up for 10 years, allowing information on changes in chronic respiratory system over the years to be collected (Abbey et al. 1991, 1993). Approximately 7,000 Seventh-Day Adventists, chosen because they do not smoke, were interviewed in 1977. Those who had lived at least 11 years in areas of Southern California identified as having high or low pollution were compared on the basis of chronic respiratory status (Hodgkin et al. 1984). Residents of the higher pollution area had a 15 percent higher rate of chronic obstructive pulmonary disease than residents in the lower pollution area after adjusting for age, sex, occupational exposure, race, and past smoking history. This included chronic bronchitis, asthma, and emphysema. Euler et al. (1987) used the same population sample and found a statistically significant association between past TSP exposure and chronic respiratory disease. Past TSP exposure was based on residence zip-code history. As noted earlier, however, analysis of data from this cohort did not generally observe mortality effects with TSP. The follow-up of the original sample included 4,000 of the original participants. Separate, statistically significant associations between chronic (11-year) TSP exposure and both airway obstructive disease and chronic bronchitis were found.

Summary

Table 7.5 presents a summary of the results discussed in this and the previous chapter (Chapter 6). Several effects have been seen in both acute and chronic studies. Table 7.5 presents ranges of effect estimates relating particulate exposure (PM_{10}) to various health end points. These effect

T A B L E   7 . 5

Approximate Range of Estimated Effects Measure as Percent Change in Health Endpoint per 10 µg/m³ Increase in PM_{10} for the Different Basic Study Designs

Health Endpoints	Acute Exposure		Chronic Exposure	
	Population-Based	Cohort-Based	Population-Based	Cohort- or Sample-Based
Mortality	Total: 0.5–1.5 Resp: 1.5–4.0 Cardio: 0.5–2.0		Total: 0–5	Total: 3–9 Cardiopulmonary: 5–9 Lung cancer: 0–9
Respiratory Health Care	Hospit. Admit: 0.5–4.0 Emergency Visits: 0.5–3.5			
Decrease in Lung Function		FEV: 0.05–0.35 PEF: 0.04–0.25		Lung function 0–2
Respiratory Symptoms, Disease		Lower: 0–15 Upper: 0–7 Cough: 0–25 Asthmatic attacks: 1–12		Emphysema, Chronic bronchitis or cough 10–25
Restricted Activity	Grade school absences: 1.0–4.0	Restricted activity days: 1.0–5.0		

Adapted from Pope 1996.

estimates are expressed as percent change in the end point per 10 $\mu g/m^3$ increase in pollution. The studies discussed here and others have observed human health effects associated with chronic exposure to respirable particulate air pollution. Population-based cross-sectional studies that evaluated spatial distributions of mortality and air pollution have observed associations between mortality and particulates. The associations between sulfate or fine particulate fraction of air pollution and mortality is stronger and more statistically significant than between SO_2 or Total Suspended Particulates (TSP). The population-based studies have been criticized partly because they were not able to control directly for individual differences in cigarette smoking and other risk factors.

We deliberately refrain from making a quantitative comparison of the various studies. The numbers in the population (ecological) studies depend upon the independent variables to include in the analysis. If collinear variables, particularly other pollutants which vary collinearly with PM_{10} are included, the effect can be made to vanish (Lipfert 1990). While this may be considered implausible, the proof comes from the cohort studies. The two cohort studies cannot be directly compared either. Although in each study the health of individual people were studied, and their individual habits were noted, their exposure and hence dose still came from a community based monitor. In the six cities study, care was taken to have a monitor at a "representative" location. In the ACS study, the EPA monitoring network was used. It is likely that some of the EPA monitors were close to the sources leading to a high exposure estimate, and a lower measured coefficient of air pollution related mortality. For these and other reasons we merely state a range in Table 7.5.

Recent studies that could adjust for individual differences in other risk factors, however, have observed that long-term exposure to respirable particulate air pollution was associated with small deficits in lung function and higher risk of chronic respiratory disease and symptoms. Two recent prospective cohort studies observed increased mortality risks associated with air pollution—even after directly controlling for individual differences in age, sex, race, cigarette smoking, and other risk factors. The present epidemiological studies cannot distinguish between $PM_{2.5}$ and sulfates (SO_4) as the causative agents in air pollution related mortality, as has been emphasized by Lipfert and Wyzga (1995a, b). Both $PM_{2.5}$ and sulfates are good proxies for combustion related air pollution. The hypothesis that the observed mortality and morbidity effects are primarily due to combustion source particulate air pollution needs further laboratory testing.

Although the biological linkages remain poorly understood, the results of the acute and chronic exposure studies are complementary. In all epidemiologic studies there is the concern that the observed association is due to confounding, that is, that it results from a risk factor that is correlated with both exposure and mortality but is not adequately controlled for in the study design and analysis. Important potential confounders in cross-sectional studies, such as unaccounted for differences in occupational exposure or socioeconomic variables, are not likely to be confounders in daily time-series studies because such factors are unlikely to change daily in correlation with air pollution levels. The fact that both daily time-series studies and cross-sectional studies observe qualitatively coherent associations between respirable particulate pollution and mortality further supports the hypothesis that this pollution is an important risk factor for respiratory disease and cardiopulmonary mortality. However, it must be noted that while the cross-sectional studies, if real, must include the effects observed in the time-series studies, the inverse is not the case.

In conclusion, current epidemiologic evidence suggests that respirable particulate air pollution, at levels common to many urban and industrial areas in the United States, contributes to human morbidity and mortality. Long-term, repeated exposure increases the risk of chronic respiratory disease and the risk of cardiorespiratory mortality. Short-term exposures can exacerbate existing cardiovascular and pulmonary disease and increase the number of persons in a population who become symptomatic, require medical attention, or die. The pattern of cardiopulmonary health effects associated with particulate air pollution that has been observed by epidemiological studies is the strongest evidence of the health effects of this pollution. Nevertheless, the epidemiological studies have important limitations that stem largely from the use of people who are living in uncontrolled environments, and who are exposed to complex mixtures of particulate air pollution.

In addition to providing limited information about biological mechanisms, current epidemiological studies provide relatively meager information about the relative health impacts of various constituents of air pollution including the possible differential impact of indoor and outdoor exposures. Furthermore the relationships between the relative importance of chronic versus acute exposures remains unclear. Much of the recent epidemiological effort has focused on effects of acute exposure, primarily because of the relative availability of relevant time-series data sets. However, the effects of chronic exposure may be more important in terms of overall public health relevance. Such research is also needed to provide a better understanding of susceptible populations. For example, individuals susceptible to serious effects of acute exposure may only be those with existing respiratory and/or cardiovascular disease; but, a much larger segment of the population may eventually be seriously effected by chronic, long-term exposure.

8

Airborne Particles and Respiratory Disease: Clinical and Pathogenetic Considerations

Mark Utell and Jonathan Samet

Introduction

As noted in Chapter 1, there is no doubt that the well-chronicled and dramatic air pollution episodes of 40 and more years ago, like the London fog of December 1952, had a major impact upon health. Laws and regulations enacted and promulgated in Europe and the U.S. since then reduced the major air pollution concentrations, and there were no such large episodes from the 1970s on. The new series of reports (since 1970) that showed an association between particulate air pollution and mortality discussed in detail in Chapters 6 and 7 have been both unanticipated and controversial. They show associations at levels of particulate pollution at least an order of magnitude lower than measured during the earlier episodes—levels lower than the current standard in the United States. The findings have potentially profound implications for regulations governing outdoor air quality; in the United States, the findings imply that the present standard for particulate matter does not provide an adequate margin of safety, as required by the U.S. Clean Air Act. Moreover, the suggestion by some analysts that there is a non-threshold type of relationship, would contradict the assumptions made in this act that an absolutely safe level is possible.

In Chapters 6 and 7 the studies, reviews and critiques of these studies of mortality and complementary studies of morbidity were discussed and appear to be robust. We place these findings into a clinical perspective, addressing mechanisms by which particles could adversely affect potentially susceptible groups within the population including infants and the elderly, and persons with advanced heart and lung diseases. We begin by considering the prevalence rates of these possibly susceptible groups and their characteristics. We then review the findings of the clinical studies, involving controlled exposures of volunteers to inhaled particles. We end with a discussion of potential pathogenic mechanisms.

Populations At Risk

Several lines of evidence suggest that persons in the population at risk from inhaled particles are those with severe heart and lung diseases and perhaps elderly people. In the London fog of 1952, the proportion of deaths attributed to heart and lung diseases increased during the dates of the fog (Brimblecombe 1987). A similar pattern has been found in the contemporary studies as well (Schwartz 1994). Additionally, because heart disease is the leading cause of death in the United States, any effect of particulate air pollution on total mortality would be expected to reflect at least an adverse impact on persons with heart disease.

The principal diagnostic labels assigned to this potentially susceptible group in the population by virtue of having chronic heart or lung disease would include coronary artery disease or ischemic heart disease inclusive of persons with a history of myocardial infarction or coronary-artery bypass surgery, chronic obstructive pulmonary disease (COPD), and asthma. Persons with coronary artery disease have atherosclerotic narrowing of the coronary arteries which deliver blood to the heart. Persons with COPD have physiologically significant impairment of lung function, most often from underlying emphysema and airways narrowing caused by smoking. Asthma has been defined as an inflammatory disorder of the airways with accompanying airways hyperresponsiveness and the clinical manifestation of variable airflow obstruction (DHHS 1991). Other groups considered to be potentially susceptible include persons affected by pneumonia or other severe respiratory infections, and infants and the elderly in general.

Estimates have been made on the sizes of these potentially susceptible groups. The American Lung Association (1993) has published estimates of their numbers in its publication, *Breath in Danger II*. For particulate matter, the groups assumed to be at risk in the report include pre-adolescent children ($\leq$ 13 years old), the elderly ($\geq$ 65 years old), and persons with pre-existing respiratory disease including COPD and asthma. Population data from the 1990 Census were used at the county level. Estimates of the population having COPD and asthma were based on the National Health Interview Survey; these national data were applied at the county level. Non-attainment was based on 1991 data from the Environmental Protection Agency.

In 1991, 74 cities and counties, with a total population of 40,208,738, were in non-attainment for PM_{10}. These cities and counties included 8,468,492 pre-adolescent children, 4,581,242 elderly persons, 610,874 children less than 18 years of age with asthma, 1,068,385 adult asthmatics, and 2,227,190 persons with COPD. These categories are not exclusive and cannot be totaled. If persons with coronary heart disease were also considered at risk from PM_{10} are also considered at risk, than an additional 1,600,000 persons, or about 4 percent of the total population, would be added. While these estimates should be considered only as approximate, they signal a basis for public health concern. On the other hand, the numbers of persons in these susceptibility groups who are truly fragile and vulnerable to premature death are likely to be substantially smaller than the American Lung Association's estimates. Furthermore, the purported susceptibility of preadolescents has not been established. The assumption of the preadolescents' susceptibility has been based on anticipated increased lung doses of pollutants because of outdoor activity.

Lung Dosimetry

Particle dosimetry in the respiratory tract has a central position in considering mechanisms as it addresses the key issue of sites of deposition, independent of specific particle composition. Dosimetry information is also needed for extrapolation of findings from animal studies to humans. Dosimetry models can also be used to understand the influence of compromised lungs in altering regional lung dose and lung defenses against inhaled particles.

From the perspective of health-related actions of aerosols, interest is limited to particles that can at least penetrate into the nose or mouth and particularly to particles that deposit on respiratory tract surfaces. The respiratory tract in humans can be divided into three major regions on the basis of structure, size, and function: the extrathoracic (ET) region that extends from just posterior to the external nares to the larynx; the tracheobronchial region (TB) defined as the trachea to the terminal bronchioles where proximal mucociliary transport begins; and the alveolar (A) or pulmonary region including the respiratory bronchioles and alveolar sacs.

Although deposition of inhaled particles in specific regions depends on multiple factors, including the aerodynamic properties of the particle (primarily size), airway anatomy, and breathing pattern, several generalizations can be made. Particles larger than 15 μm are effectively filtered out in the nose and nasopharynx (ET). These relatively large particles tend to settle rapidly because of impaction and gravitational forces. "Clearance" refers to the dynamic properties in both airways and alveoli that remove particles physically from the respiratory tract. The actual amount of the substance in the respiratory tract at any time is called retention.

Particles between 1 μm and 20 μm diameter are commonly encountered in the work place and ambient air. Submicron particles are perhaps the most numerous in the environmental air. Particles in the nanometer size, the so-called "ultrafine" range, are of concern because of the large number of particles per unit mass as well as potential toxicity (Oberdoster et al. 1995). These spherical, non-hygroscopic particles deposit in the respiratory tract by three principle mechanisms: inertial impaction, gravitational sedimentation, and Brownian diffusion. In humans, the turbinates of the nose and glottic aperture in the larynx are areas of especially high air velocity, abrupt directional changes, and turbulence, and efficiently remove large particles (>5.0 μm) in the ET region by impaction (Figure 8.1). Gravitational sedimentation occurs when a particle settles out of an airstream due to the force of gravity. For particle diameters greater than 0.5 μm, sedimentation and impaction are the primary deposition mechanisms. In the pulmonary region, gravitational sedimentation is the principal mechanism of particle deposition with deposition probability increasing with increasing residence time. For particles less than 0.5 μm in diameter, Brownian diffusion becomes a dominant mechanism. Deposition by diffusion depends on particle diameter; smaller particles diffuse more rapidly. As particles decrease in size to the ultrafine range (< 0.01μm), they begin to behave more and more like a highly reactive gas diffusing rapidly towards the airway walls. Deposition of small particles (< 0.5 μm) on surface walls can be enhanced by electrostatic forces resulting from surface charges on particles. Finally, the deposition of hygroscopic particles depends on the extent of growth in the humid conditions of the respiratory tract. Ferron, Heyder and Kreyling (1985) have examined the effect of particle growth on total deposition. For a 1.0 μm dry NaCl aerosol, total deposition is 80% compared with 20% for the same size non-hygroscopic aerosol.

The above generalizations regarding typical particle deposition in normally breathing adults are subject to great variability. Deposition into specific regions of the respiratory tract can be influenced by changes in respiratory flow rates, respiratory frequency, and tidal volume. Consequently, the activity level of an individual may result in a change in the mode of breathing (mouth vs. nasal breathing) and can significantly alter regional as well as total respiratory tract deposition of inhalable particles. Mouth breathing results in decreased removal of particles by the upper

FIGURE 8.1

Schematic Representation of Four Major Mechanisms Causing Particle Deposition

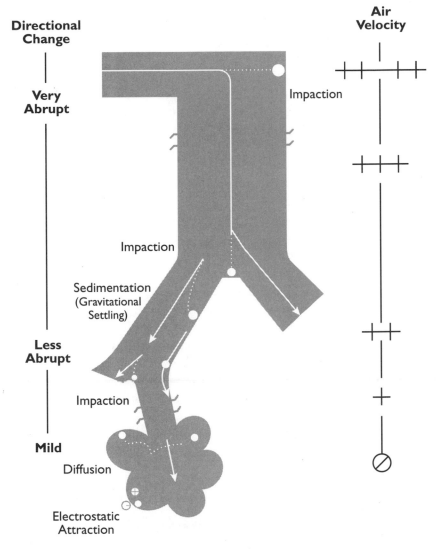

Airflow is signified by arrows, particle trajectories by dashed lines.

respiratory tract allowing deeper penetration into the lung. Kim, Lewars and Sackner 1988) have demonstrated greater deposition of particles in subjects with lung disease; more recently, model simulations of compromised lungs show greater numbers of particles deposited per alveolus in compromised compared with non-compromised lungs (Miller et al. 1995). However, the contribution that differential deposition and clearance of particles might make to observed morbidity and mortality has not been determined.

Mechanistic Considerations

How could inhaled particles increase mortality on a short-term basis? A variety of mechanisms have now been postulated (Table 8.1) (Bates 1992, Dockery and Pope 1994, Schlesinger 1995). These mechanisms are not necessarily exclusive and they are overlapping in scope. Bates (1992) introduced the concept of coherence in assessing the health effects of air pollution. He proposed that there are plausible relationships among indices of the adverse effects of air pollution and also proposed three mechanisms as to why respiratory and cardiovascular mortality might rise together during air pollution episodes; 1) acute bronchitis and bronchiolitis may be incorrectly diagnosed as pulmonary edema; 2) increased lung permeability from air pollutants could precipitate pulmonary edema in persons with myocardial damage and increased left atrial pressure; and 3) the imposition of acute bronchiolitis or pneumonia caused by air pollution on preexisting heart disease could precipitate heart failure.

Any mechanism should be consistent in its time scale with the time frame on which the association between daily counts of mortality and air pollution measures has been observed, e.g., one or two days. Thus, acute inflammation with increased permeability and increased airways resistance could plausibly underlie a short-term effect. Increased susceptibility to respiratory infection, by contrast, would not be anticipated to increase mortality immediately.

If these mechanisms are to be considered as underlying the association of particulate air pollution with mortality, then it is also necessary to

---

TABLE 8.1

Proposed Mechanisms Underlying Association Between Particulate Pollution and Mortality

- Increased airways permeability
- Impaired host defenses
- Alveolar inflammation
- Exacerbation of chronic lung disease
- Specific toxicities

invoke the companion concept of the existence of pools of susceptible persons who are sufficiently fragile to have their deaths advanced by pollution exposure. These persons presumably would represent the most severely affected persons with chronic lung and heart diseases and particularly fragile elderly and children, such as those with bronchopulmonary dysplasia.

Review of the Evidence from Controlled Human Exposures

Introduction

These potential mechanisms by which particulate air pollution could affect mortality are best explored using controlled human exposures of volunteers who are representative of those considered at risk. Such carefully-controlled, quantitative studies of exposed humans, often referred to as "clinical studies," offer a complementary approach to epidemiologic investigations for understanding the effects of inhaled pollutants in populations (Utell and Frampton 1993). Human clinical studies employ laboratory atmospheric conditions that can replicate the exposure of interest from ambient pollution. In the laboratory setting, clinically relevant effects can be documented and markers of injury, reflective of pathogenetic mechanisms, can be assessed. Protocols can be designed to characterize exposure-response relations. In addition, the controlled environment of the exposure chamber provides the opportunity to examine interactions among components of a pollutant mixture or between pollutants and other factors, such as exercise, humidity or temperature.

To the extent that individuals with chronic respiratory and heart diseases can participate in exposure protocols, potentially susceptible populations can be studied. However, clinical studies have limitations; for practical and ethical reasons, studies are limited to small groups which may not be representative of larger populations, to exposures of short duration, and to pollutant concentrations that are expected to produce only mild and transient responses. Additionally, participants in clinical studies are volunteers and not likely to be representative of those at highest risk for dying from the underlying disease. In fact, studies of asthmatics have been shown to restrict the study population to those with mild disease (Samet 1989). Endpoint assessment invariably includes pulmonary function, but biological specimens may be collected to assess markers of injury. With healthy volunteers, relatively invasive procedures, including fiber optic bronchoscopy, may be part of the protocol.

Controlled clinical studies may address both healthy volunteers and individuals with underlying cardiopulmonary diseases. Subjects are typically characterized by age, gender, race, and lung function. Volunteers are usually classified as "healthy" by the absence of allergies, often documented by skin testing, and the lack of hyperreactive airways assessed by inhalation challenge tests. Within this rubric of healthy, adolescent, elderly normal, and "smoker," subgroups have been studied in various protocols. Healthy volunteers are typically able to perform vigorous exercise for extended periods and are usually able to tolerate the more invasive techniques such as lavage of the lungs through a fiberoptic bronchoscope, bronchoalveolar lavage.

Other susceptible groups that have been recruited to participate in clinical studies include asthmatics, individuals with allergies or acute upper respiratory infections, and subjects with COPD or coronary artery disease. For research and clinical purposes, asthmatics can be characterized by the degree of nonspecific airways responsiveness to methacholine or carbachol, presence or absence of allergy (skin tests or IgE levels), use of medications, severity of symptoms, and degree of airway obstruction assessed by pulmonary function tests.

Exercise performed either on a treadmill or bicycle ergometer is often a component of the challenge protocol. Exercise enhances the pollutant dose both by increasing ventilation and thereby the amount of the pollutant inhaled and by causing a switch from nasal to oral breathing; oral breathing has the effect of bypassing the nose which is efficient in removing particles and gases and thereby protecting the lower respiratory tract. In addition, the effect of exercise on airway drying may enhance the response to pollutants. While it is clear that minute ventilation during exposure is an important determinant of the magnitude of change in selected physiological measures, the influence of exercise pattern (continuous versus intermittent) on pulmonary function responses is less certain. The impact on pulmonary function of exercising at different intensities during pollutant exposures has been reviewed by Horvath (1985).

Ideally, the exposure protocols should be double-blind and use a crossover design with sodium chloride for the control aerosol. In a cross-over design, the same subjects are exposed to both the challenge and control aerosols. The investigator, the technician, and the subject should be unaware of whether the subject is receiving the true exposure or a control exposure. This strategy eliminates a potential for observer bias and avoids relaying clues to volunteers regarding anticipated responses.

This section summarizes recent controlled human exposure studies on particulate air pollution. These studies were reviewed previously by Utell (1985) and more recently by the U.S. EPA Acid Aerosols Issue Paper

(EPA 1989). The few reports of controlled exposures to diesel, carbon black or other particles are reviewed. We emphasize studies in individuals with underlying lung disease, recognizing that responses are typically defined by changes in mechanics; however, findings from healthy volunteers, especially alterations in defense mechanisms or cellular responses, are also considered, if relevant. There have not yet been any studies that have involved exposure of persons with heart disease to particles.

Diverse aerosols are produced by air pollution, gas phase reactions and dispersion of organic dust, e.g., tree resins, pollens, decaying vegetation and spores. Combustion processes concomitantly release unconverted liquid and solid fuels and wind erosion continually disperses terrestrial and marine surface materials. Of this mixture of natural and anthropogenic aerosols, clinical studies have tended to examine primarily the latter category, especially inorganic sulfates and nitrates, which play a prominent role in "acid rain." We consider the evidence separately for soluble and insoluble particles.

Soluble particles

In the atmosphere, the major acid sulfate species include ammonium sulfate $[(NH_4)_2SO_4]$, ammonium bisulfate (NH_4HSO_4), and sulfuric acid (H_2SO_4). In the laboratory, pulmonary responses of normal and asthmatic subjects have been assessed following exposure to each of these acids. Nitrate particles will not be considered in this review since they have not been found to provoke either symptoms or functional decrements in clinical studies at concentrations less than 1,000 $\mu g/m^3$ (EPA 1989), far higher than the range of interest in considering the epidemiologic data on particles.

Studies of healthy volunteers

Controlled experimental exposures have been used to examine the respiratory effects resulting from the inhalation of acidic aerosols, with measured outcomes limited primarily to symptoms and airway function. Although exposures to concentrations of H_2SO_4 aerosols below 1,000 $\mu g/m^3$ generally do not alter airway function of normal subjects (Utell and Morrow 1983, 1984) observed an increase in throat irritation and airway reactivity to carbachol inhalation in normal volunteers 24 hours after exposure to 450 $\mu g/m^3$. No change in airway reactivity was detected immediately after exposure. Slowing of mucociliary clearance in small airways began at H_2SO_4 concentrations as low as 100 $\mu g/m^3$ (Spektor and Yen 1989); the duration of the slowing increased with hours of exposure.

Only one study has been performed to examine the effects of H_2SO_4 aerosols on host defense mechanisms at the alveolar level (Frampton et al. 1992). Non-smoking volunteers were exposed for two hours to an aerosol of approximately 1,000 $\mu g/m^3$ H_2SO_4 or NaCI with intermittent exercise, in a random double-blind fashion. Bronchoalveolar lavage was performed 18 hours after exposure in order to detect evidence of an inflammatory response, change in alveolar cell subpopulation, or changes in alveolar macrophage function, all components of host defense. When compared with NaCI, exposure to H_2SO_4 did not increase the number of polymorphonuclear leukocytes in the lavage fluid. The percentage of T lymphocytes decreased in association with H_2SO_4 exposure, but not significantly. Antibody-mediated cytotoxicity of alveolar macrophages increased in association with H_2SO_4 exposure. Significant changes were not found in release of superoxide anion of inactivation of influenza virus *in vitro*. The investigators concluded that brief exposures to H_2SO_4 aerosols at 1,000 $\mu g/m^3$ did not cause an influx of inflammatory cells into the alveolar space, and no evidence was found for alteration in alveolar antimicrobial defenses 18 hours after exposure.

As with sulfur dioxide (SO_2), asthmatic subjects have been found most susceptible to the effects of acidic aerosol exposure although different laboratories have found differing threshold exposure concentrations. In general, however, studies of adult asthmatics have failed to demonstrate alterations in lung function at levels below 200 $\mu g/m^3$. Utell and co-workers (Utell et al. 1983) exposed asthmatics to H_2SO_4, NH_4HSO_4, $NaHSO_4$, and a control NaCI aerosol at concentrations of 100, 450, and 1,000 $\mu g/m^3$. Following exposures to the 450 and 1,000 $\mu g/m^3$ concentration aerosols for 16 minutes, specific airway conductance decreased in relation to the acidity of the aerosol, supporting the hypothesis that airway effects are related to acidity rather than to the sulfate ion. More prolonged exposures to H_2SO_4 aerosols have also been performed. With ten-minute exercise periods every 30 minutes, a two-hour exposure to 100 $\mu g/m^3$ H_2SO_4 aerosol resulted in a small reduction in flow rates; high ambient levels approach this concentration. The response to H_2SO_4 was maximum after the first 45 minutes and then airway function recovered and returned towards baseline. The effect did not appear to be progressive over time. Respiratory ammonia was identified as a factor influencing responses to sulfuric acid aerosols; by reducing the level of endogenous respiratory ammonia, airway responses to inhalation of 350 $\mu g/m^3$ aerosols in exercising asthmatics were enhanced (Morrow et al. 1994). This finding provided further evidence that aerosol acidity significantly affected bronchoconstriction caused by inhalation of sulfate aerosols.

Functional decrements have been observed in adolescent asthmatics at levels as low as 68 µg/m³ for 40 minutes (Koenig, Covert and Pierson 1989), suggesting that adolescent asthmatics are more sensitive to the effects of acidic aerosols than adult asthmatics. The apparent difference in sensitivity of adult and adolescent asthmatics may also be due to selection, differences in aerosol sizes or exposure protocols. However, the data show that adolescent asthmatics respond to concentrations of H_2SO_4 aerosols at an order of magnitude lower than normal subjects. In these studies, young asthmatics showed functional decrements at exposure levels near peak outdoor levels in the Northeastern U.S. Field studies in summer camps of both normal and asthmatic children reported decrements in pulmonary function during pollution episodes that included increased levels of acidic aerosols (Raizenne et al. 1989), reinforcing concern that children and adolescents may be particularly susceptible to effects of acidic atmospheres.

Volunteers with chronic obstructive lung disease (COPD)

Based on the epidemiologic observations and on their compromised respiratory status, subjects with COPD are considered to be potentially at high risk for mortality and morbidity from particles. To determine whether inhalation of low-level H_2SO_4 aerosol induces alterations in lung function in COPD patients, older volunteers (mean age 62 years) were exposed to 90 µg/m³ H_2SO_4 aerosols in an environmental chamber for two hours (Morrow and Utell 1995). Subjects were classified as having COPD on the basis of dyspnea on exertion, obstructive airways disease (mean forced expiratory volume in one second [FEV_1] = 1.4 liters or 53% predicted, and mean ratio of FEV_1 to forced vital capacity [FVC] = 0.56) and a lack of response to bronchodilators. In contrast to the findings in persons with asthma, the volunteers with COPD did not have larger drops greater in pulmonary mechanics in response to H_2SO_4 than to sodium chloride, the control aerosol. Subjects with COPD, presumably the most vulnerable subpopulation, demonstrated virtually no change in the rates at which air could be exhaled, even with periods of intermittent mild exercise during the exposure.

The findings of these studies provide evidence that asthmatic patients may experience adverse effects on airway function at relevant high ambient levels of soluble particles. Collectively, these data demonstrate that asthmatics do manifest significant, albeit small, reductions in their performance during moderate physical activity after inhaling acidic aerosol concentrations close to high ambient levels. For asthmatics, the irritant potency of sulfate aerosols appears related to acidity per se. Inhalation of the more acidic sulfates produces the most significant bronchoconstriction while exposure to less acidic sulfate aerosols causes no significant change in lung function. Other findings suggest that the amount of titrable acidity in an aerosol is a determinant of these adverse pulmonary effects (Fine and Gordon 1987). In any case, the decrements in lung function are relatively small after exposure to acid particles, and they are non-progressive, and mitigated by ammonia neutralization. Individuals with COPD do not appear to respond to particle inhalation with broncho-constriction or respiratory symptoms.

Insoluble particles

Inhalation of insoluble particles has been used primarily as a tracer to examine long-term clearance kinetics from the human lung and not to assess inherent toxicity. In a study reported by Bailey and Fry (1982), subjects inhaled 10 breaths of an aliquot of 25 µl fused aluminosilicate particles (FAP) suspended in ethanol. Monodisperse 1.2 µm and 3.9 µm diameter particles were labeled with radioactive tracers. Following inhalation, clearance was followed for over 200 days. Approximately 8% of 1.2 µm and 40% of 3.9 µm particles cleared within 65 days. Overall retention of the remaining material showed half-times averaging 320 days, with considerable intersubject variation. Approximately 10 other studies examining long-term clearance rates in man have been performed with particles such as iron oxide, manganese oxide, or polystyrene; clearance half-times have generally been faster than 320 days (Bailey and Fry 1982). Effects on symptoms and lung function were not found in these studies, presumably because of the low particle concentrations and very short exposure times.

Monodisperse Teflon particles labeled with [111]I have been used to study regional deposition in healthy and asthmatic volunteers. In similar types of studies, deposition of diethyl hexyl sebacate particles of less than 1.0 µm has been examined in subjects with obstructive and restrictive lung diseases (Anderson and Wilson 1990). Particle loads were achieved after four to 10 breaths and inhalation of the experimental aerosols probably required less than 1 minute. Although the deposition and retention patterns vary depending on particle size and presence of underlying airway obstruction, no effects on lung function parameters were reported. The failure to detect clinical responses may reflect the minimal exposure to only four to 10 breaths of aerosol and the small sample size.

Few clinical studies of respiratory toxicity have been performed with insoluble particles. In one recent controlled exposure study, healthy and asthmatic volunteers inhaled respirable carbon particles (Anderson and Avol 1992). Four exposure scenarios were used: 1) clean air; 2) 0.5 μm H_2SO_4 aerosol at 100 μg/m^3; 3) 0.5 μm carbon aerosol at 250 μg/m^3; and 4) 250 μg/m^3 carbon plus 100 μg/m^3 H_2SO_4 aerosol generated from fuming sulfuric acid. Electron microscopy demonstrated that nearly all the acid in group 4 became attached to carbon particle surfaces, and that most particles remained in the submicron group range. All exposures were for one hour with alternate 10-minute periods of exercise and rest. Symptoms and lung function were measured before, during and after exposure while bronchial reactivity to methacholine was measured post-exposure. Analyses were performed for effects of H_2SO_4 or carbon, separately and combined, on all outcome measures. The investigators concluded that for both healthy and asthmatic subgroups, mean changes in lung function measures associated with the experimental pollutants were small and of no clinical significance. In persons without lung disease, forced expiratory function measurements did not show significant variation associated with exposure to carbon and/or sulfuric acid. Likewise the changes in lung function for the asthmatic groups did not suggest a significant adverse effect of the pollutants, separately or combined, in comparison with the effect of clean air.

Finally, Sandstrom and Rudell (1991) examined the bronchoalveolar inflammatory response to inhalation of diesel exhaust. Diesel exhaust from an idling diesel engine was diluted with air and introduced into an exposure chamber. Median concentrations in the breathing zone were 3 x 10^6 particles/cm^3, 3.7 ppm NO, 1.6 ppm NO_2, 27 ppm CO, and 0.3 mg/m^3 formaldehyde. Exposures were performed for one hour and included moderate exercise on a bicycle for 10-minute periods alternating with rest. Lavage was performed 18 hours after exposure and demonstrated an increase in neutrophils in the bronchoalveolar but not the bronchial portion of the lavage. Phagocytosis of opsonized yeast cells in vitro by macrophages from the bronchoalveolar lavage was significantly altered. Since exposures to pollutant gases such as SO_2 or NO_2 alone have typically not induced an acute inflammatory response, the investigators speculated that the responses may have been caused by particles or hydrocarbons in the diesel exhaust.

Synthesis

Insoluble particles have been used primarily for measuring deposition and clearance kinetics from the human lung. Unfortunately, too few clinical studies have been performed with either carbon or diesel particles to allow meaningful conclusions in normal subjects and none have involved volunteers with COPD.

Pathophysiologic Mechanisms

Clinical pathophysiologic mechanisms

A role for particles in causing new cases of disease cannot be considered as a mechanism to explain the association of particle concentrations with variation of daily mortality counts. Although particulate matter could be linked to the genesis of asthma, chronic bronchitis, or other airways diseases, the time course of effect likely would require many years and would not be compatible with the epidemiologic finding of association between mortality and day-to-day variation in mortality counts.

Review of the potential mechanisms by which present ambient concentrations of inhaled particles could be associated with mortality highlights gaps in the toxicologic evidence now available. Particle dosimetry in the respiratory tract is an excellent starting point for considering biological plausibility of the epidemiologic findings, as it addresses key issues from a perspective independent of specific particle composition. When different ventilatory regions of the lung are compromised with respect to their ventilatory capacity, as in persons with asthma, COPD, or congestive heart failure, those regions of the lung that are unaffected may receive a disproportionately high dose of particles. Consequently, those remaining healthy regions of the lung may be injured and the lung's reserve capacity further compromised. However, an increase of ambient particle concentrations by 20–40 $\mu g/m^3$, the range of variation typical in many urban locations, would translate into a relatively small increase in peripheral lung particle deposition. From a pathophysiologic perspective, it seems unlikely that the resulting particle burden could worsen ventilation-perfusion ratios in either healthy or injured lung regions to the point of producing clinically significant hypoxemia, i.e., a degree of hypoxemia sufficient to cause pulmonary edema from left ventricular failure, increased permeability, or malignant arrhythmia (Table 8.1).

Similar considerations argue against exacerbation of respiratory infections from deposited particles. Alternative explanations for the relationship between particles and mortality include an increased likelihood of respiratory infections in individuals with COPD or asthma. Particle exposure could increase susceptibility to infection from bacteria or respiratory viruses, leading to an increased incidence of, and death from pneumonia. However, although pneumonia can result in death within 24 hours of onset, serious infections of the lower respiratory tract generally develop and evolve over days and weeks; these time relationships are not consistent with the observed association on a daily basis. Moreover, hospital admissions should increase in parallel with mortality and the widespread availability of ventilatory support would tend to further blunt any immediate effect of particle exposure on pneumonia mortality. If pollutant exposure increased susceptibility to specific infectious diseases, it should be relatively easy to detect marked differences in the incidence of such diseases in communities with low vs. high particulate concentrations, given appropriate control for other contributing factors. To date, no such relationships have been observed, although there has been little research on specific etiologic agents in relation to variation in pollutant concentrations. Finally, although the increased work of breathing could undoubtedly lead to increased mortality in individuals with chronic lung disease, no specific link between particle exposure and work of breathing has been identified.

Evidence of a dose-response relationship, increasing risk of an adverse effect with increasing exposure, bolsters the argument for causality. The epidemiologic data are indicative of dose-response relationships for morbidity and mortality measures. These data sets have largely been analyzed with regression techniques that assume a linear relationship between the response variable and the predictor variables. The regression coefficients describe the association between the air pollution exposure variables and the morbidity and mortality indexes (Table 8.2). There is thus abundant evidence from the epidemiologic studies of increasing risks from particles with increasing ambient concentrations as assessed by linear regression models. However, the linear dose-response model represents one biologically plausible representation of the relationship between particle exposure and health risk; alternative models e.g., curvilinear and threshold have not received equal attention.

TABLE 8.2

Potential Mechanisms Underlying the Association of Particulate Air Pollution with Mortality

- ■ Increased susceptibility to infection from impaired host defenses
- ■ Airways inflammation leading to impaired gas exchange and hypoxia
- ■ Provocation of alveolar inflammation by ultrafine particles with release of mediators that exacerbate underlying lung disease and increase blood coagulability
- ■ Increased lung permeability leading to pulmonary edema
- ■ Precipitaton of heart failure in those with chromic cardiac disease by acute bronchiolitis or pneumonia induced by pollution

Little evidence of dose-response relationships can be found in the clinical toxicologic literature, even though the ranges of concentrations exceed those usually experienced by the general population. Even at high particle concentrations in susceptible subpopulations, acidic aerosols produce only small decrements in lung function.

Toxicological mechanisms

One general mechanism of interest is pulmonary inflammation. Potential mechanisms for induction of an inflammatory response have been described for: (1) ultrafine particles, (2) transition metal ions and (3) aerosol acidity.

Recently, Seaton et al. (1995) have proposed that the mechanism of particle-induced injury involves the production of an inflammatory response by ultrafine particles (< 0.02 μm diameter) in the urban particulate cloud. As a result, mediators are released capable of causing exacerbation of lung disease in susceptible individuals and increased coagulability of the blood. Several hematological factors, including plasma viscosity, fibrinogen, factor VII, and plasminogen activator inhibitor not only predict cardiovascular disease but also rise as a consequence of inflammatory reactions. In support of Seaton's proposed mechanism is the observation in an animal model that ultrafine particles cause greater inflammation than larger particles of the same substance (Oberdoster et al. 1995). These investigators demonstrated that inhalation of Teflon particles in the ultrafine range between 0.01 μm and 0.03 μm for 15–30 minutes by rats resulted in the development of acute pulmonary hemorrhagic edema with a high influx of inflammatory PMNs in the lung. A concentration of about 10^5 particles/cm^3 of these Teflon fume particles is equivalent to a mass concentration of 9 μg/m^3. Teflon fumes consist of vapor-phase constituents in addition to the ultra-fine particle phase, and toxicity could be related to the ultrafine, vapor-phase component or both. In these experiments, fluoride concentration approximated 10 ppm whereas hydrogen fluoride levels as high as 1300 ppm have produced toxic effects in the upper respiratory tract without significant changes in the peripheral lung. Further more, other investigators have demonstrated that removal of the particle phase by filters and exposure of rats to the vapor phase only did not lead to the toxicity found with total Teflon fumes. To exclude the possibility that oxygen-derived radicals on the surface of these particles may cause the highly toxic response, particles were also generated by using Teflon in an argon gas atmosphere which caused the same degree of toxicity. Therefore, given the essentially inert nature of Teflon, one would conclude that ultrafine particles, in and of themselves, are capable of eliciting the acute inflammatory responses.

The hypothesis that freshly-generated ultrafine particles when inhaled as singlets at very low mass concentrations can be highly toxic to the lung is supported by their high deposition efficiency in the lower respiratory tract, their large numbers per unit mass, and their increased surface areas available for interactions with cells. Based on the predictive lung deposition models for inhaled particles, ultrafine particles inhaled as singlets of a size of about 0.02 µm have the highest deposition efficiency in the alveolar region of the lung in humans. Up to 50% of inhaled ultrafine particles of this size are deposited there. Assuming a resting minute ventilation of 8 l/min and an exposure concentration of 1×10^5 particles/cm^3, about 80 particles would be deposited in one hour per alveolus in a human lung having 3×10^8 alveoli per lung. While this is a large number of particles, it represents a tiny mass; for example, with 0.02 µm particles of unit density, 2.4×10^6 particles/cm^3 are required to achieve 10 µg/m^3, whereas for 2.5 µm particles only about 1 particle/cm^3 gives the same mass concentration (Oberdoster 1996).

Another suggestion is that surface coating of ambient particles with transition metals (e.g., iron) will lead to an increased inflammatory reaction after phagocytosis of these particles due to the generation of more toxic oxygen-derived radicals. (Tepper et al. 1994) instilled particles with surface-complexed iron (Fe^{+3}) and produced inflammation in rat lungs 96 hours after instillation, as indicated by increased polymorphonuclear leukocytes, eosinophils and total protein in lavage fluid. The investigators hypothesized that the surface-complexed iron generate hydroxyl radicals in the lung and that these radicals have acute lung toxicity.

A third toxicologic hypothesis, (noted in Chapter 5) has been that acidic particles or a coating of particles with acid (e.g., H_2SO_4) could be responsible for particle effects. Laboratory data in guinea pigs by Chen et al. (1992) and Amdur and Chen (1989) indicate that low levels of H_2SO_4 coated onto carrier particles resulted in inflammatory responses in the conducting airways of the animals.

Despite the increasing effort to identify a mechanism by which low concentrations of particles cause cardiopulmonary toxicity, to date we are left with only speculative hypotheses. Studies have not been performed with relevant ultrafine ambient particles and models involving instillation of particles with or without metals or acids may induce toxicity not typical of inhalation. Each of these approaches warrants more rigorous testing.

Clinical mechanisms

Underlying heart and lung disease may affect patterns of particle deposition. The obstructive lung diseases, asthma and COPD, characteristically result in inhomogeneity of ventilation within the lung. Heart failure, through its effect on airways function, may also affect the distribution of ventilation. When some ventilatory regions of the lung are compromised with respect to their ventilatory capacity, the remaining healthy regions of the lung can receive a disproportionately high dose of particles and thus further compromise the lungs' reserve capacity. However, an increase of ambient particle concentrations of 20–40 $\mu g/m^3$, typical of the range of excursions in U.S. cities, would translate into relatively small increases in peripheral lung particle deposition; from a pathophysiologic perspective, it seems unlikely that this particle loading could worsen ventilation-perfusion ratios in either healthy or abnormal lung regions to the point of producing life-threatening hypoxemia.

There is a similar lack of plausibility in attempting to relate exacerbations of respiratory infections to increased particle loads. Alternative explanations for the relationship between particles and mortality include an increased likelihood of respiratory infections in individuals with COPD or asthma. Particle exposure could increase susceptibility to infection with bacteria or respiratory viruses, leading to an increased incidence of, and death from pneumonia. However, although pneumonia can rarely result in death within 24 hours of onset, serious infections of the lower respiratory tract generally develop and evolve over days and weeks, and would not explain effects on daily mortality. Moreover hospital admissions should increase and the widespread availability of ventilatory support would tend to blunt further any immediate effect of particle exposure on pneumonia mortality. If pollutant exposure increased susceptibility to specific infectious diseases, it should be relatively easy to detect the consequent marked differences of such diseases in communities with high versus low particle concentrations, with appropriate control for other confounding factors. To date no such relationships have been observed. Finally although the increased work of breathing could undoubtedly lead to increased mortality in individuals with chronic lung disease, no specific link between particle exposure and work of breathing has been established.

Summary

In considering the biological plausibility of this new evidence on adverse effects of particles, we emphasize the following principles: consistency with clinical observations, consistency with other observed effects of air pollutants on humans, and consistency with toxicological investigations using animal models. The most perplexing observation in regard to these criteria is that of excess daily mortality associated with 24-hour average particulate concentrations as low as 50 $\mu g/m^3$. Although there is no question as to the plausibility of a causal relationship between higher levels of particulate exposure and excess mortality, as observed, for example, in the London smog episodes with particulate concentrations as high as 4000 $\mu g/m^3$, uncertainty about causality increases when this relationship is extended down to concentrations as low as 50 $\mu g/m^3$. Although individuals at risk for mortality from particles would be expected to spend more time indoors and the contribution of ambient particles to personal exposure would be further reduced, unless only fine particles are responsible for which high penetration factors are achieved.

Nevertheless, the epidemiologic observations show a consistent relationship between particle concentration and mortality. Moreover, no immediate alternative explanation exists for these findings. The epidemiologic data appropriately identify the same susceptible populations at greatest risk as would be anticipated clinically; however, no data on exposure patterns of these susceptible groups are available. The impact of outdoor concentrations on total personal exposure of susceptible populations is also unknown.

Neither clinical experience nor review of the literature identify a direct pathophysiologic mechanism that can be to explain the relationship between inhaled particles and mortality. There are limitations in the toxicologic data base. Human toxicologic studies directly relevant to ambient particles are sparse and fail to replicate ambient particle mixtures. None of the human and few of the animal studies have yet used particle generation systems that reflect the complexity of ambient particles. It seems unlikely that there is a highly toxic and still unidentified particle that fails to produce even an inflammatory response in normal airways but when deposited in injured airways can cause death. Any postulated mechanism must therefore show how responses to small to be inflammatory can nonetheless when combined with other situations increase the likelihood of death slightly but enough to be visible in a large population.

The recent animal toxicologic studies provide a possibility for new insights for future research in human toxicology. Studies with real-world particles with surface complexed iron (Tepper et al. 1994), ultrafine Teflon particles (Oberdoster et al. 1995), sulfuric acid-coated ultrafine metallic particles (Amdur and Chen 1989) or fine carbon particles (SPH) provide interesting models linking a specific component of real-world particulate matter with frank inflammatory effects in animals. Novel approaches provide opportunities to identify mechanisms of injury including characterization of the role of mediators, the identification of neurotransmitters, and an understanding of the subtleties of immune suppression. Such techniques could eventually uncover mechanisms by which these particles alone or in a complex with metals could produce pulmonary edema, arrhythmia or exacerbation of sever obstructive airways disease. Currently, such mechanisms remain highly speculative, and largely theoretical.

A research agenda should be developed and implemented as a basis for a more informed interpretation of the epidemiologic evidence and the development of future policy. Given the lack of acceptance of biologic mechanisms for the observed associations of particle concentrations with morbidity and mortality, unidentified limitations of the statistical models used for analysis should not be dismissed. Perhaps subsequent reanalyses of the data, possibly including pooled analyses, may help resolve the dilemma. As we have previously suggested (Utell and Samet 1993), the framework for interpreting the epidemiologic finding will be inadequate until these needed data are available.

9

Modeling of Air Pollution Impacts: One Possible Explanation of the Observed Chronic Mortality

John Evans and Scott Wolff

Introduction

In Chapter 7, the statistical relationships between air pollution and mortality have been described in some detail. If taken at face value, and extrapolated linearly to low levels of exposure, these relationships imply that there is an excess of 50,000 premature deaths occur in the U.S. each year due to current levels of ambient particulate matter. Despite the fact that over the past two decades the evidence of a statistical *association* has become more compelling, this still does not prove *causality* and some scientists and others question the legitimacy of the observed relationships on grounds that it is biologically *implausible*. What biological mechanism explains, or even could explain, the results found by cross sectional and time series mortality studies?

As explained earlier in Chapter 8, there are in fact a number of biological mechanisms which *could* be responsible for the effect. These include the impairment of host defenses, increased airway permeability, increased airway and alveolar inflammation, and exacerbation of chronic lung disease. In the current chapter we take one of the arguments advanced by Utell and Samet a bit further and explore the quantitative plausibility of one possible mechanism that might describe the results of the cross-sectional studies. To be quantitatively plausible, we believe that we must be able to construct a mathematical model of a process, which violates no biological laws or data, that is able to describe a large fraction—perhaps 75% or more—of the observed increase in mortality. If the mechanism suggested was only able to explain, for example 1% of the mortality rate, it might not be wrong, but it would be irrelevant. More specifically, we examine the possibility that the chronic effect appearing in the cross sectional studies is due to a reduction in lung function, and that this reduction in lung function is caused by air pollution. We therefore examine the relationships between air pollution, lung function and mortality.

It is well established that exposure to air pollution can impact lung function—i.e., that it can accelerate the rate of decline of lung function as we age (Xu et al. 1991). Independently it has been shown that individuals with reduced lung function face increased risk of death—i.e., that the level of lung function is a good predictor of mortality (Beaty et al. 1985). Thus, several authors have argued that the impacts of air pollution on lung function could in principle lead to increased mortality in those so affected (Evans et al. 1984, Dockery et al. 1993, Dockery and Pope 1994, Crawford and Wilson 1996).

In addition to the potential health impacts posed by air pollution, cigarette smoking also contributes to an increased risk of mortality. The relative loss of life expectancy in smokers and non-smokers resulting from air pollution is illustrated, very schematically, in Figure 9.1. The figure

FIGURE 9.1

Schematic of Lung Function vs. Age Showing Loss of Life Expectancy (LOLE)

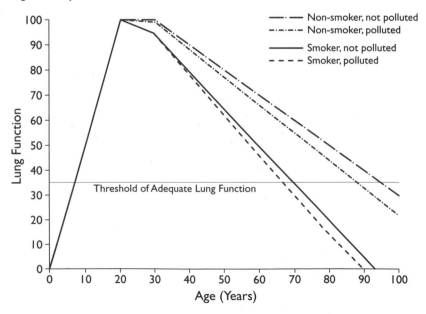

plots lung function vs. age, showing how it is expected to fall steadily from a maximum at age 20–30 to a level where there is inadequate lung function. In healthy persons lung function remains adequate throughout life, and never falls below a threshold lung function necessary for survival. It is well known that smoking measureably reduces lung function, and this is plotted. In the absence of other causes of death, smoking, in the example shown, brings lung function to the dangerous level at 70 years instead of 95 years—a Loss of Life Expectancy (LOLE) of 25 years. The addition of air pollution reduces life expectancy by 6 years for a non-smoker and 3 years for a smoker. Competing causes of death reduce both these figures. The model suggests that this potential impact will be noted primarily in the infirm populations whose lung function has already decreased for other reasons and will appear as an increase in mortality risk among the aged, or simply as a loss of life expectancy.

This chapter addresses the quantitative nature of the above relationship, allowing for all the competing causes of death, by presenting a modeling approach to examine the possibility that the current low levels of particulate air pollution in the U.S. could be responsible for the mortality seen in cross-sectional epidemiology studies. We presented some initial background for this model in an earlier publication (Evans et al. 1982). This analysis utilizes data from the Six Cities Study of Air Pollution and Lung Function (Dockery et al. 1988, Xu et al. 1992) on age-specific baseline lung function and data from the Framingham Heart Study (Sorlie 1989) on the relationship between lung function and mortality. We consider whether the relationship required to produce this mortality excess is consistent with the experimental data currently available.

Method of Calculation

Operationally the model estimates the impact of air pollution on mortality by comparing the mortality experience of two hypothetical cohorts that are identical except with respect to their exposures to particulate air pollution—one cohort is exposed to chronic low levels (1 $\mu g/m^3$) of particulate air pollution and the other receives no exposure. The cohort not exposed to particulate air pollution provides the model's estimate of baseline age-specific lung function and mortality. By comparing the lung function and resultant mortality in this cohort with that in the unexposed cohort, we assess the possible mortality impact of air pollution. Mortality is estimated separately for each age group from age 0 to 100. The total mortality for each population is defined as the sum of the annual age-specific deaths estimated to occur throughout a single year.

A life table approach is at the center of the modeling analysis. In a life table, the probability of surviving from age 0 to age x is simply the product of the age-specific survival probabilities:

$$s_x = p_0 {}^* p_1 {}^* \cdots {}^* p_{x-1} \qquad (9\text{-}1)$$

where s_x is the probability that an individual will survive from age 0 to age x, and $p_0, p_1, \ldots, p_j, \ldots, p_{x-1}$ are the age-specific annual survival probabilities— i.e., the probability of surviving from his j^{th} birthday to his age $j+1^{st}$ birthday.

Using this basic framework, we have utilized data from the Framingham Heart Study to model the relationship between lung function and the age-specific annual survival probabilities (Sorlie et al. 1989). Table 9.1 presents the probablity of dying within a specific 10-year period for males estimated from the Framingham Study (Sorlie et al. 1989). This relationship between lung function and the annual probability of survival is expressed as:

$$p_j = f\left(j, L_j\right) \qquad (9\text{-}2)$$

where j is the age (yr), L_j is lung function at age j normalized for body height (L/m^2) and f is the function relating age and age-specific lung function to annual survival probability.

These relationships have the general form:

$$p_j = \left(1 - \exp\left(-a_j - b_j {}^* L_j\right)\right)^{0.1} \qquad (9\text{-}3)$$

TABLE 9.1

Ten Year Probabilities of Death (for Males) as a Function of Age and Lung Function

Age (Yr.) Start of 10-yr. Interval	Lung Function, FEV_1, Normalized for Height(L/m^2)		
	0.10–0.69 (mean = 0.4)	0.70–0.99 (mean = 0.85)	1.00–1.59 (mean = 1.3)
55–59	0.19	0.21	0.16
60–64	0.52	0.30	0.17
65–69	0.56	0.40	0.27
70–74	0.59	0.55	0.37
75–79	0.72	0.63	0.66
80–84	0.88	0.70	0.69

Data are 10-year death rates from Exam 13 of the Framingham Heart Study (Sorlie et al. 1989).

where p_j is the age-specific annual survival probability, L_j is the age-specific lung function (L/m^2) and both a_j and b_j are age-specific coefficients. Table 9.2 presents estimates of the parameters a_j and b_j derived from the Framingham Heart Study (Exam 13) by regression analysis. Other parameters are provided in this table as well.

To complete the analysis, it is necessary to model the relationship between age and lung function in both cohorts—those exposed to chronic particulate air pollution, and those not exposed. Because smoking has such a pronounced impact on both lung function and on mortality, it is necessary to stratify the analysis—first by analyzing the relationships between air pollution, lung function and mortality for non-smokers, then re-analyzing these same relationships for smokers, and finally by computing the impact on a mixed population of non-smokers and smokers.

The first relationship that we examine is the age-dependence of lung function. Lung function, which declines with age in response to various problems including the decreasing elasticity of lung tissues, is typically characterized on the basis of physiological measurements such as FEV_1 (forced expiratory volume in one second) or FVC (forced vital capacity). It is now common to include a standard measure such as FEV_1 after

TABLE 9.2

Estimates of the Mortality Lung Function Parameters

Age, j	Parameter Value			
(yr)	a_j	b_j	c_j	d_j
50–54	1.100	0.693	0.583	-
55–59	1.100	0.693	0.487	2.03
60–64	0.625	0.693	0.489	2.03
65–69	0.351	0.693	0.383	2.03
70–74	0.122	0.693	0.319	1.08
75–79	0.040	0.300	0.371	1.08
80–84	0.040	0.300	0.271	1.08

c_j is the fraction of smokers in the specified age group at Exam 13 of the Framingham Heart Study (O'Connor, 1996).

d_j is the relative risk of death from all causes among smokers after adjusting for lung function, taken from the results of Exam 13 of the Framingham Heart Study (O'Connor 1996).

Note: Although the data from the Framingham study does not include information for individuals in the age groups 85–89, 90–94, and 95–99, we assume that the parameter values appropriate for the 80–84 age group can also be applied to these older individuals.

adjustment for an individual's height (FEV$_1$/ht^2). Our analysis uses data adjusted for height, and where necessary we use a nominal adult male height of 1.73 m to scale the data.

Baseline Lung Function among Non-Smokers

An essential parameter to be defined in the model is the potential effect that age has on lung function. Lung function declines with increasing age. The decrement in lung function is thought to start after age 25, and first becomes clinically apparent at approximately age 40.

The model follows the defined physiologic parameters of the aging process by assuming that lung function does not decrease with age until an individual reaches age 26. After this age, the model assumes there is an age-specific decrease in lung function for each age and each level of natural variability.

Baseline age-specific lung function among non-smokers has been obtained from the work of Dockery and Xu (Dockery et al. 1988; Xu et al. 1992). The basic form of the relationship given by Dockery in his Table 4 (for men) is:

$$L_j = L_{50} - 0.0347 * (j - 50) - 0.000204 * (j - 50)^2 \qquad (9\text{-}4)$$

where L_j is the lung function (FEV$_1$, normalized for height $[L/m^2]$) at age j, and L_{50} is lung function at age 50.

It is well known that there is a great deal of heterogeneity even in age-specific lung function. For example, Dockery et al. have estimated that the distribution of lung function as measured by FEV (among 50 year old males) is approximately normal with a median FEV$_1$ value of 3.63 liters, and a standard deviation of 0.50 liters. Our analysis accounts for this heterogeneity in lung function by dividing the population into subgroups on the basis of their baseline lung function at age 50. Specifically, we follow separately the life experience of seven subgroups—one with median lung function, and six others with median plus (or minus) one, two and three standard deviations of baseline lung function. The mortality experience of the whole population is then computed by integrating the separate experiences of these seven subgroups. It will be seen that including the tails of the distribution is essential for obtaining a reasonably accurate value of the effect of air pollution.

Table 9.3 presents selected values of the estimated age-specific lung function values in units of FEV$_1$ (liters). These same data are presented graphically in Figure 9.2.

TABLE 9.3

Baseline Lung Function by Age and Variability among Non-Smokers Without Air Pollution Impacts

Fraction of Population	Lung Function, FEV_1 (L)			
	Age (yr)			
	25	50	75	100
Median +3 S.D.	5.88	5.14	4.15	2.90
Median +2 S.D.	5.38	4.64	3.64	2.39
Median +1 S.D.	4.87	4.13	3.14	1.89
Median	4.37	3.63	2.63	1.38
Median -1 S.D.	3.87	3.13	2.13	0.88
Median -2 S.D.	3.36	2.62	1.63	0.38
Median -3 S.D.	2.86	2.12	1.12	0.00

FIGURE 9.2

Lung Function vs. Age

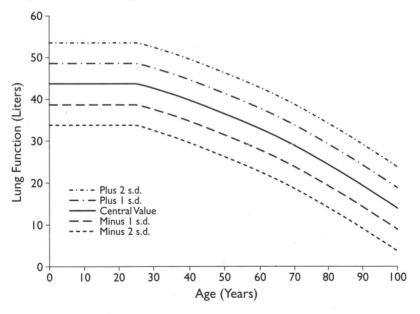

Baseline Mortality among Non-Smokers

Using the data on baseline age-specific lung function in conjunction with the relationships between lung function and mortality, it is possible to construct a baseline life table for this population. The model was implemented using a Lotus 1-2-3 Release 4.0 spreadsheet. Selected values of age-specific baseline mortality estimates for non-smokers (without air pollution impacts) are given in Tables 9.4 and 9.5.

The life expectancy (at birth) of the population may be estimated as:

$$e_0 = s_0 + s_1 + \ldots + s_{100} - \frac{1}{2} \tag{9-5}$$

The life expectancy of each of the seven susceptibility groups was computed using equation (9-2) to define the relationship between survivorship and annual survival probabilities; equation (9-3) to relate these annual survival probabilities to age-specific lung function (with the parameters a_j and b_j chosen for non-smokers); and equation (9-4) to characterize the baseline age specific lung function values appropriate for non-smokers in each of the groups.

The impact of baseline lung function on age-specific survival probabilities on life expectancy is readily apparent. Our analysis indicates that a person with median baseline lung function has a life expectancy at birth of 73.9 years and a 45% chance of surviving to age 75. In contrast, a person with superior baseline lung function (median + 3 sd) has a life expectancy at birth of 77.2 years and a 58% chance of surviving to age 75. Whereas an individual with inferior lung function (median - 3 sd) has a life expectancy at birth of only 70.3 years and a 29% chance of surviving to age 75.

T A B L E   9 . 4

Baseline Cumulative Survival Probability by Age among Non-Smokers Without Air Pollution Impacts

Fraction of Population	Probability of Surviving to Age x Age (yr)				Life Expectancy at Birth (yr)(e_j)
	25	50	75	100	
Median +3 S.D.	1.00	0.99	0.58	0.042	77.2
Median +2 S.D.	1.00	0.99	0.54	0.030	76.1
Median +1 S.D.	1.00	0.99	0.50	0.021	75.0
Median	1.00	0.99	0.45	0.013	73.9
Median -1 S.D.	1.00	0.99	0.40	0.007	72.7
Median -2 S.D.	1.00	0.99	0.35	0.003	71.5
Median -3 S.D.	1.00	0.99	0.29	<0.001	70.3
Entire Population	**1.00**	**0.99**	**0.45**	**0.012**	**74.7**

Deaths associated with a decrease in lung function not assumed to occur until age 50.

TABLE 9.5

Baseline Age-Specific Mortality among Non-Smokers Without Air Pollution Impacts

Baseline Lung Function	Population in Group	Number of Deaths at Specified Ages					
		Age (yr)				All	(%)
		25	50	75	100		
Median +3 S.D.	620	0	4	37	3	597	96.3%
Median +2 S.D.	6,060	0	46	369	23	5,900	97.4%
Median +1 S.D.	24,170	0	207	1,490	71	23,742	98.2%
Median	38,300	0	368	2,372	79	37,881	98.9%
Median -1 S.D.	24,170	0	262	1,490	32	24,025	99.4%
Median -2 S.D.	6,060	0	74	367	4	6,043	99.7%
Median -3 S.D.	620	0	9	36	0	620	100.0%
Total Population	100,000	0	969	6,160	153	98,807	98.8%

The model estimates the total stationary population as 7,384,644 individuals. The number of deaths per year is calculated as 98,807. Therefore the crude mortality rate is estimated as: (98,807)/(7,384,644) or 1,338 per 100,000 per year.

Effect of Cigarette Smoking on Lung Function and Mortality

The experiences of smokers are quite different that those of non-smokers. Epidemiologic studies that compare death rates for smokers to non-smokers indicate that smoking has a dramatic effect on mortality (Mattson et al. 1987). Since other life-style factors which could significantly affect mortality are controlled for in these studies, the observed difference in mortality in smokers and non-smokers can be directly attributed to smoking.

Although, the majority of this increased mortality in smokers is attributed to cardiovascular effects, cancer and stroke, respiratory function can also be affected. Lung function declines more rapidly among smokers than among non-smokers and this may lead to increased risk of death at every age (see Figure 9.1). In addition, synergistic (i.e. additive) effects resulting in potential exponential increases in mortality due to smoking may exist in the exposed populations, however, these effects have not been included in our analysis.

The health effects model for smokers assumes that an individual begins smoking at age 25 and continues smoking for the rest of his life. A smoking rate of 1.3 packs/day is also assumed in the model corresponding to a medium/heavy smoker. Since smoking begins at age 25, a maximum estimate of 97.5 pack-years is possible for an individual surviving until 100 years of age.

In our model, smoking impacts life expectancy in two ways—first, it exacerbates the rate of decline of lung function, and second, it acts to elevate the baseline age-specific probabilities of death. We use a relationship given by Dockery et al. (1988) to assess the impact of smoking on lung function:

$$\frac{d\ FEV_1}{dt} = -0.0074 PY_j - 0.123 SM_j \qquad (9\text{-}6)$$

where $d\ FEV_1/dt$ is the rate of change of lung function with age (L/yr), PY_j is the cumulative pack years smoked by age j, and SM_j is a dummy variable taking the value 1 for current smokers and 0 otherwise. We adjust the baseline relative risk of death from all causes (conditional on age specific lung function) using data from Table 9.2 giving the relative risk of mortality for smokers as 2.03 for the age groups 50–59 and 1.08 for ages 70–74.

Table 9.6 presents the lung function estimates for smokers included in the seven susceptibility groups. Tables 9.7 and 9.8 give the age-specific survival estimates and life expectancies for smokers. Note that the estimated impact of smoking on life expectancy is approximately 7.5 years— a value similar to the amount of time required to smoke the approximately 700,000 cigarettes by each individual included in the analysis.

The Potential Impact of Air Pollution on Lung Function

In our model, the impact of air pollution on mortality is indirect. Air pollution exposure is assumed to accelerate the rate of decline of lung function and in this way to indirectly increase the rate of mortality and reduce life expectancy.

To simplify the analysis, we have estimated the impact of chronic (lifelong) exposure to an increment of 1 µg/m³ of airborne particulate matter. Further, we assume that the increment in the rate of decline of lung function with age is proportional to the level of air pollution exposure, so that:

$$\frac{d\ FEV_1}{dt} = -k * A \qquad (9\text{-}7)$$

TABLE 9.6

Baseline Lung Function by Age and Variability among Smokers Without Air Pollution Impacts

Fraction of Population	FEV_1 (L)			
	Age (yr)			
	25	50	75	100
Median +3 S.D.	5.72	4.74	3.50	2.01
Median +2 S.D.	5.22	4.24	3.00	1.51
Median +1 S.D.	4.71	3.73	2.50	1.01
Median	4.21	3.23	1.99	0.50
Median -1 S.D.	3.70	2.72	1.49	0.00
Median -2 S.D.	3.20	2.22	0.98	0.00
Median -3 S.D.	2.70	1.72	0.48	0.00

Smoking assumed to begin at age 25.

TABLE 9.7

Baseline Cumulative Survival Probability by Age among Smokers Without Air Pollution Impacts

Fraction of Population	Probability of Surviving to Age x				Life Expectancy at Birth (yr) (e_i)
	Age (yr)				
	25	50	75	100	
Median +3 S.D.	1.00	0.98	0.37	0.008	71.1
Median +2 S.D.	1.00	0.98	0.32	0.004	69.8
Median +1 S.D.	1.00	0.98	0.26	0.002	68.5
Median	1.00	0.98	0.21	0.001	67.1
Median -1 S.D.	1.00	0.97	0.16	<0.001	65.8
Median -2 S.D.	1.00	0.97	0.11	<0.001	64.5
Median -3 S.D.	1.00	0.97	0.06	<0.001	63.1
Entire Population	**1.00**	**0.98**	**0.21**	**0.001**	**67.2**

Deaths associated with a decrease in lung function not assumed to occur until age 50.

where the rate of decline of lung function (k) is given in L/yr per $\mu g/m^3$ and the level of air pollution, A, is expressed in terms of the annual average concentration of particulate matter ($\mu g/m^3$).

Our literature review identified no recent estimates of k for adults. Our colleagues at the Harvard School of Public Health have recently published a study that included decrements of lung function estimates in children living in 22 U.S. and Canadian communities (Spengler et al. 1996,

TABLE 9.8

Baseline Age-Specific Mortality among Smokers Without Air Pollution Impacts

Baseline Lung Function	Population in Group	Number of Deaths at Specified Ages					
		Age (yr)				All	(%)
		25	50	75	100		
Median +3 S.D.	620	0	10	30	1	615	99.2%
Median +2 S.D.	6,060	0	107	286	6	6,033	99.6%
Median +1 S.D.	24,170	0	482	1,073	71	24,125	99.8%
Median	38,300	0	866	1,556	8	38,280	99.9%
Median -1 S.D.	24,170	0	620	865	0	24,170	100%
Median -2 S.D.	6,060	0	177	180	0	6,060	100%
Median -3 S.D.	620	0	21	14	0	620	100%
Total Population	100,000	0	2,283	4,005	86	99,902	99.9%

The model estimates the total stationary population as 6,714,105 individuals. The number of deaths per year is calculated as 99,902. Therefore the crude mortality rate is estimated as: (99,902)/(6,714,105) or 1,488 per 100,000 per year.

Raizenne et al. 1996). Figure 9.3 presents the results of the regression analysis utilizing mean estimates of the concentrations of two particulate matter sizes in 22 cities: $PM_{2.1}$ (k = -0.004 L/yr per $\mu g/m^3$) and PM_{10} (k = -0.003 L/yr per $\mu g/m^3$) vs. FEV_1. Estimates of the lower-bound 95% confidence interval of k for the two particle sizes range from: $PM_{2.1}$ (k = -0.0006 L/yr per $\mu g/m^3$) and PM_{10} (k = -0.00008 L/yr per $\mu g/m^3$). It is likely that children may be more susceptible to the effects of air pollution than adults. Since we are concerned with the chronic effect of air particulates on adults it is best to utilize the lower bound estimates of k. For simplicity in the calculation, we have chosen a value of k = -0.0001 L/yr per $\mu g/m^3$ to use in the analysis. We realize that other estimates of k may be available that could be evaluated in future analyses.

The next step in the model is to consider a population of identical individuals exposed to a chronic air particulate concentration of 1 $\mu g/m^3$ throughout the entire year. The incremental effect that this low level of chronic air pollution has on the age-specific loss of lung function is estimated. Potential deaths are tabulated for the individual age groups when the total lung function estimate (baseline—pollutant effect) is decreased to the point that the potential survival of the individual is threatened. These potential deaths associated with the baseline and pollutant effects are summed across all age groups and subtracted from the baseline mortality rate estimate in order to derive a crude mortality rate

FIGURE 9.3

Lung Function Estimates for Children in 22 U.S. and Canadian Communities

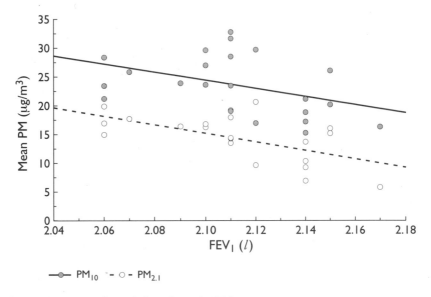

Source: Raizenne et al. 1996, Spengler et al. 1996.

based on air particulates assumed at a standard concentration of 1 μg/m³. The k value of -0.0001 L/yr per μg/m³ is utilized in the model. This potential impact of air particulates on lung function in non-smokers is added to the baseline effects calculated above to estimate a total effect on lung function and mortality.

Table 9.9 presents the age-specific mortality estimates for the baseline and pollutant effects in non-smokers and smokers. The crude mortality rate for non-smokers exposed to pollutant effects is estimated as 1,338.43 deaths/year per 100,000 individuals. This compares with the baseline predicted mortality estimate of 1,338.01 deaths/year per 100,000 individuals. The difference in the two mortality estimates for non-smokers is calculated as 0.42 deaths/year per 100,000 individuals exposed to 1 μg/m³ of air particulates chronically throughout the year. For smokers, the baseline crude mortality rate is a bit higher, 1,487.95 deaths/year per 100,000 individuals, and the rate in the pollution exposed cohort of smokers is also higher, 1,488.42 deaths/year per 100,000 individuals, but the estimated incremental impact of exposure to air pollution is relatively similar at 0.47 deaths/year per 100,000 individuals.

TABLE 9.9

Estimated Impact of Chronic Exposure to 1 µg/m³ Particulate Air Pollution on Mortality Among Non-Smokers and Smokers

Population	Baseline Lung Function	Life Expectancy (yr)		
		Baseline	Pollution	Change
Non-Smokers	median + 3 sd	77.195	77.180	0.015
	median + 2 sd	76.107	76.092	0.015
	median + 1 sd	74.994	74.978	0.016
	median	73.857	73.842	0.015
	median - 1 sd	72.701	72.685	0.016
	median - 2 sd	71.526	71.510	0.016
	median - 3 sd	70.331	70.315	0.016
	All Never-Smokers	**74.730**	**74.715**	**0.015**
Smokers	median + 3 sd	71.105	71.085	0.020
	median + 2 sd	69.795	69.776	0.019
	median + 1 sd	68.473	68.454	0.019
	median	67.143	67.124	0.019
	median - 1 sd	65.810	65.790	0.020
	median - 2 sd	64.473	64.453	0.020
	median - 3 sd	63.122	63.102	0.020
	All Smokers	**67.207**	**67.186**	**0.021**

Note that these risks correspond to losses of 0.015 yr * 365 day/yr or 5.5 days of life expectancy at birth among non-smokers, and 0.021 yr * 365 day/yr or 7.7 days among smokers.

The Integrated Impact of Air Pollution on Mortality

The number of predicted deaths associated with particulate air pollution has been estimated above for both smokers and non-smokers in the health effects model. An estimate of the total impact on a specific population of interest can be derived by knowing the percentage of non-smokers and smokers in the population.

The fraction of smokers in the U.S. population has been decreasing in recent years, but for several earlier decades was relatively constant with approximately 50% of men classified as current smokers. Utilizing this approximate value, the mortality in a mixed population of half non-smokers and half smokers would be approximately 0.45 deaths/year per 100,000 individuals per µg/m³ of particulate matter.

Discussion

The coefficients derived from cross-sectional mortality studies discussed in Evans, Tosteson and Kinney (1984) were 0.34 deaths/year per 100,000 persons per µg/m³ of TSP particulate matter, which is approximately 0.61 deaths per yea r per µg/m³ of PM_{10}. These are typical of the values discussed in Chapter 7. These values are highly consistent with our preliminary estimates based on the assumption that a 1 µg/m^3 level of total particulate matter increases the rate of decline of lung function by approximately 0.0001 L per year.

Although there are no reliable studies of the rate of decline of lung function caused by chronic exposure to air pollution, the values that we have selected are physiologically plausible. However, the rate of decline of lung function that is necessary to produce the observed mortality is too small to be definitively detected in any study completed so far.

This work suggests that quite small absolute impacts of air pollution on lung function could in fact be responsible for the mortality observed in cross-sectional studies. Thus, it is quite possible to produce 50,000 premature deaths each year in the U.S. due to relatively low levels of ambient particulate levels without needing to invoke physiologically implausible mechanisms.

We here recapitulate the assumptions of the model. Firstly that air pollution makes an irreversible change in the lung which reduces lung function in proportion to the integrated air pollution. Secondly that although this reduction in lung function may be unimportant for a young healthy adult, it can accentuate other problems in the weak and infirm or merely elderly. Since the effect of the air pollution is indirect with an intermediate observable effect (lung function), the model predicts that any other cause of reduction in that intermediate effect (lung function) will produce ailments in a population in the same proportions. This is a deduction that is, in principle, verifiable.

We emphasize an important feature of this model and class of models. The basic medical process postulated—that inadequate lung function can lead to death—has a threshold. Yet in a population composed of people of various degrees of lung function, including the infirm and the aged and those who unfortunately smoke tobacco, a small incremental risk is calculated for a small increment in pollution.

This model *only* addresses the chronic effects of continuous exposure to air pollutants. It *does not* address the acute response immediately following a peak of exposure as shown in the time series studies discussed in Chapter 6, although an extension of this model should enable it to do so.

We suggest that an important way of making progress in this field is to make models such as this one to derive numerically verifiable predictions and try to verify them. For example the age structure of the deaths and the distribution of diseases in a population should be calculated and checked for overall consistency.

Hill (1965) suggested a number of attributes of a calculation, that would assist in inferring causality from an association between an effect and a postulated cause. These will be discussed in full in Chapter 10. One of them was "biological plausibility." We suggest that the mechanisms listed in Chapter 8, and the detailed calculations on one postulated mechanism here, make the case for biological plausibility (but not for biological proof).

Nonetheless it is self evident that not all experts in air pollution and public health are convinced that low concentrations of fine particles, either per se or because of acid or heavy metal coatings or both, cause adverse effects on health. Even fewer members of the public and politicians are so convinced. We echo a sentiment quoted on page 214 of the first edition of this book, "unfortunately there has been very little work on models of air pollution related mortality...." We suggest that development and testing of quantitative general models such as this are likely to be important next steps in preparing an adequately convincing proof. Such development is long overdue.

10

Conclusion:
Policy Implications:
The National Dilemma

Richard Wilson and John Spengler

The Evidence

In the preceding chapters we have discussed the evidence that airborne particulates severally or in combination, from stationary or mobile fossil fuel-burning facilities, cause a human health hazard at 1996 ambient air pollution levels. The epidemiological data compare human death rates and morbidity rates with air pollution variables. As the data have developed over the last 30 years, the correlations have appeared to be better with Total Suspended Particulates (TSP) rather than with sulphur dioxide, with PM_{10} rather than TSP, and with fine (<2.5 µm) particulates ($PM_{2.5}$) rather than the coarse fraction. Unfortunately measurements of fine particles are rare. Those less than 10 microns (PM_{10}) have only recently (since 1985) been measured extensively and smaller ones not at all in most urban air sheds.

Data on animals, discussed in Chapter 5, which are tentatively extrapolated to humans, had suggested for many years that particles—probably sulfuric acid particles—were more irritant than SO_2 per se. At the time of the first edition of this book, the epidemiological studies, admittedly only population based, ecological, studies, seemed to be in accord with this tentative conclusion from the animal studies; the association with air pollution was greater for sulfates or TSP than for SO_2 itself. This suggested the idea that combustion products, particularly perhaps the complex combustion products of coal, were responsible for the observed adverse health effects. Recent animal studies discussed in Chapter 5 have confirmed that bronchial problems are caused by acid, particularly sulfuric acid aerosols, alone or complexed with metals. Some scientists have suggested that it is the H+ ion itself that is the proximate cause of the health problems. Yet nitric acid seems less irritant to animals than sulfuric acid. Moreover, acid particulates are likely to be neutralized when they penetrate indoors.

But here the epidemiological studies seem to have a slight divergence. This immediately leads to a puzzle. The time-series data of acute mortality and morbidity presented in Chapter 6, seem to give us a coefficient of air pollution related mortality in Los Angeles, where nitrogen oxides predominate among the particles, as large as that in Steubenville where sulfate particles predominate. One cohort mortality study from the population of adults followed in Harvard's 6-city study, show that ambient $PM_{2.5}$ (fine particles) and sulfate particles are stronger predictors of lower survival probabilities (higher death rates). TSP, PM_{10} and hydrogen ion concentrations all are weaker predictors. Unfortunately sulfuric acid content, or even acidity, of polluted air has not been measured extensively enough for any epidemiological refutation or confirmation of this postulate.

Another issue remains completely open. Although the time series studies of acute mortality seem definite, and the most obvious interpretation is that already ill people have their lives shortened by a comparatively short period of a month or so, there is no evidence on whether the period is a week or ten years. Moreover, the chronic studies seem to give a coefficient of mortality similar to that of the acute studies with a reduction of life expectancy counted in years. This immediately raises the question of whether the acute studies of Chapter 6 and the chronic studies of Chapter 7 are indeed measuring the same phenomenon. Resolution of this question must await future research.

Hill's Attributes

Hill (1965) in his Presidential address to the Royal Society of Medicine suggested a number of attributes of a study that would help decide whether one could proceed from a statistical association to a finding of causality. Although there are other ways of parametrizing the discussion, Hill's attributes (often glorified by calling them criteria) are widely discussed outside the usual air pollution fraternity and widely used as a "check list" by epidemiologists. It is therefore worth repeating them here:

■ Strength of the Association. If the strength were great, little other evidence would be needed. In the 1952 London air pollution incident, the death rate rose to three times the normal level within hours after the start of the air pollution increase, as shown in Figure 1.1. There was, and is, no problem of statistical accuracy. No one now questions the causality for those air pollution episodes and incidents. But causality is questioned for the effects now being claimed at lower exposures and doses where the Risk Ratio is only slightly above unity. Such a small Risk Ratio is not normally considered enough for an attribution of causality by itself so that further examination is necessary.

■ Consistency of the association. Does the same result appear at different times and places with different data analysts? The answer in general is YES. The time series data discussed in Chapter 6 show similar results in many cities of the U.S., Europe and Brazil . Some differences appear in China, where correlations with SO_2 seem stronger than with TSP, but this may be explained by considering SO_2 as a surrogate for sulfates.

■ Temporality. The exposure must always precede the disease. Inversely, if the effect is spurious, a correlation should also be found an exposure that follows the disease. Disease appears to follow exposure.

■ Dose-response. It is usual to assume that "more is worse and less is better." The dose response discussed in Chapters 6 and 7 is clearly usual. Moreover the coefficient of mortality related to concentration in the time-series studies of Chapter 6 is similar to that derived from the London air pollution incident with concentrations an order of magnitude larger.

■ Biological Plausibility. This is perhaps the most contentious of Hill's attributes. In Chapter 8 no explanation for the phenomena is found that can presently be supported, although several possibilities are suggested. But in Chapter 9 a model is postulated which can explain *quantitatively* (although not prove) the chronic health effects, and might explain the acute health effects without violating any laws. Hill specifically commented: "It will be helpful if the causation we suspect is biologically plausible. But this is a feature I am convinced we cannot demand. What is biologically plausible depends upon the biological knowledge of the day." Is Evans' and Wolff's model sufficiently plausible to satisfy Bradford Hill (or Capitol Hill)?

■ Specificity of the association. The association found in the 6 cities study and in the ACS study is with several respiratory ailments and with cardiovascular ailments but otherwise not with death rates other than respiratory. While not specific within the respiratory category, this is generally regarded as adequately specific. But a question arises which for some throws doubt on the specificity: why does cardiovascular mortality appear to be associated with ambient particles? Is the reason the same reason that smoking causes cardiovascular mortality as well as lung cancer?

■ Coherence. Does the whole body of data (including animal data and perhaps in-vitro data hang together? As Amdur (1989) pointed out in her Stokinger lecture "The Animals Tried to Tell Us" the coherence of the case for an air pollution effect related to fine, probably sulfuric acid, particles has become accepted increasingly since 1980. The coherence requires consistent evidence among related health end points. Animal data can lead us to mechanisms and suggest causative agents and exposure scenarios. They can also provide testable animal models that support clinical and epidemiological observations.

■ Experimentation. Does removal of the exposure remove the effect? This requirement is obviously met for high exposures and their effects. There has been no air pollution incident in London to match that of 1952, although in later incidents the pollution concentrations were less, people were warned to stay indoors, and the effects were far less obvious. No one has tried to stop the (smaller) exposures to fine particles discussed here, although the shut down of the steel mill in Provo, Utah has provided some data on this point. It is important to be alert to the opportunities that might be provided by war, economic changes and migration, to test the incremental changes on health.

■ Analogy. Is there a similar analogous situation which can guide us? There are few analogs to the idea that small amounts of a pollutant spread widely give small proportional effects that, integrated over a large population, appear to be large. The principal analog is in the effects of radiation at low doses. Biologically these are very different, but the disputes about the reality of a low dose effect are parallel, and the public policy implications are equally difficult.

Bates (1995) asked after a conference 10 questions that still are to some extent outstanding. We paraphrase and modify them slightly here:

■ Are the associations between PM_{10} and mortality in the time-series data robust? The answer appears to be "yes." In particular the reanalysis by Samet et al. (1995) is helpful here.

■ Can any common confounder be suggested? Confounders would be different for the time-series data of Chapter 6 and the cross-sectional series of Chapter 7. Weather and climate are the obvious confounders for the time series of Chapter 6 but the data come from several climates and temperatures. This would seem to exclude them as a common confounder. Smoking is the obvious confounder the cross-sectional studies reported in Chapter 7, but the cohab studies account for smoking but still give results that are consistent with the others.

■ Why is cardiovascular mortality related to PM_{10}? If no answer is forthcoming this might be a spurious result and suggest that the other results are spurious. This may be related to the effects of cigarette smoking.

■ Is there convincing evidence of other adverse effects of PM_{10}?

■ How does the composition of PM_{10} vary in different places or at different times? If there is such a variation, can one make a "correction" to the epidemiological data to get a weighted health effect coefficient? In the eastern United States, where there is a lot of coal burning industry, the ratio $PM_{2.5}/PM_{10}$ is higher than in San Francisco Bay area where road dust is a dominant contributor. Does that mean PM_{10} is not as bad in San Francisco Bay area?

■ Might the active particles be less than 1 micron in size? No epidemiological study yet addresses this. As noted in Table 3.1 and in the previous paragraph, the important distinction is between the fine and coarse fractions of PM_{10} which have different origins. While it may be of scientific interest to understand whether the offending particulates are small it would be irrelevant to any decision process as discussed in the next section.

■ What do we know of the effects of 10 micron and smaller particles from animal experiments? Chapters 5 and 8 provide answers to this question.

■ What future animal studies might throw light on the mechanism of effects in humans? In particular are there any suggestions of mechanisms that could be explored by epidemiologists?

■ What future epidemiological studies would be useful? One idea is that the most useful future studies will now be suggested by mathematical modeling such as that in Chapter 9.

■ Finally are the attributes of consistency, temporarility, and biological plausibility enough to draw a conclusion of causality?

■ We add an eleventh; in view of the increasing emissions of nitrogen oxides over the last decade, and the difficulty of reducing them, it is important to determine whether particulates composed of nitrates are as dangerous as other particulates as the Los Angeles acute mortality study suggests, or whether we can downplay their importance as animal studies seem to suggest.

The Decision Process

Evidence in such matters is never absolutely definite. It comes from a variety of directions and has been increasing over the last 17 years since the first edition of this book (Wilson et al. 1982) was published. The consistent picture that a public health authority should consider is that 60,000 persons might be dying prematurely of air pollution related problems in the United States each year (Shprentz et al. 1996). However, it is still argued by some that no one is dying.

This dilemma has been experienced before in other pollution problems. For example, consider the paradigm of radiation exposure. Since 1928 the International Commission on Radiological Protection (ICRP) has recommended that it be assumed that low levels of radiation may cause harm, and that the proportional relation between cancers and incident radiation dose be assumed. This assumption was, and is, made with no direct data at the low levels of concern; radiation doses, given suddenly, of 30 rem have been shown to cause cancer, yet we discuss annual natural background doses 300 times smaller (0.1 rem/yr) and increments caused by industrial activities or nuclear electric power 100 times smaller still.

In contrast, exposures to particulate air pollution at average levels of 500 µg/m^3 have been definitively shown to give rise to adverse health effects. The present (1996) U.S. air quality standard is only ten times lower than this, and there are many people exposed close to the air quality standard. It is possible to maintain, therefore, that adverse health effects from air pollution at ambient levels are more likely than adverse health effects from radiation at ambient levels, and society already has a precedent of assuming a proportional dose-response relationship (with no threshold) for handling the radiation doses.

Also with radiation an obvious anchoring point is the natural background dose; it seems intuitively reasonable to allow any extra dose that is a small fraction of the natural background and within the fluctuations of the background. The natural background for fine particulates was low before industrialization and tobacco smoking, (with the exception of the indoor air pollution from wood stoves) and particularly low for acid particulates but is now much higher over a substantial area of the U.S. and Canada and higher still throughout many urban areas of the world. Therefore natural background cannot be used for anchoring. If, as seems likely, the fine fraction of PM_{10} is responsible for the adverse health effects, there are no background measurements to anchor our understanding.

Expert Judgement

When making decisions under uncertainty society increasingly has to rely upon experts. However, this leaves open the question: who are the experts? The authors of this book, or members of a committee of the National Academy of Sciences might be called experts. Others citing a public health bias, can certainly disagree with that assumption.

Some decision makers when faced with uncertainty, a large part of which is subjective, use expert judgement elicitation. This has been done by the Nuclear Regulatory Commission for some aspects of Nuclear Reactor Safety (Wheeler et al. 1989), for Global Climate Change, and for Carcinogenic Potency assessment (Evans et al. 1994a,b; Morgan et al. 1978a,b) suggested a probabilistic approach to estimating the risk, and later (Morgan et al. 1984) attempted such a solicitation for sulfur pollution. (At that time the attribution to fine particles instead of sulfur was not widespread.) Most of these solicitations share a common feature. When a group of experts is asked about a problem, and then they discuss it among themselves, privately or at a conference, the stated uncertainty increases! This is part of a general phenomenon noted by Tversky and Koehler (1994) that subjective probability estimates are not attached to events and observations but to descriptions of events. As the description becomes more specific, and more detailed, or in technical language the problem is unpacked, the perceived uncertainty increases.

Most of the work described in this book has been completed since the last expert elicitation. It therefore seems an appropriate time to carry out another. If and when that is done, we would hope that the elicitors ask questions that appropriately "unpack" the problem so that there can be a reliable estimate of the risk.

Cost-Risk-Benefit Calculations

The most obvious and direct interpretation of the data presented here is that several (approximately four) percent of the death rate in the U.S. can be attributed to air pollution. If this interpretation is correct the effect is large and exceeds a hundredfold the sum total of all the other pollutant effects that the U.S. Environmental Protection Agency regulates. It implies that our regulatory strategies and priorities should be reconsidered. If it is desired to reduce the health risk, then new control technologies, new clean fuels, and perhaps a complete change in energy conversion technologies will be necessary to lower the exposures to a sufficient extent.

Politicians and other decision makers are increasingly turning to cost-risk-benefit calculations. If the effects were definite it would be possible to assign a "cost" to the effects on health. A number of economic studies have discussed the amount people are "Willing To Pay" to save a life that is only statistically known. As one reviewer commented none are free from objectionable features, but an average is about $4,000,000 per life (Fisher et al. 1989). With the estimate above of 60,000 premature deaths per year in the U.S. this comes to $240 billion per year. It is reasonable to assume that one quarter, or 15,000 premature deaths are the result of emissions from electricity generating stations. According to this calculus therefore we should be willing to spend $60 billion per year on changing the U.S. electrical generating system. A proper calculation would include discounting and so forth, but the sum is enough to replace all coal-fired electricity generating plants in less than 10 years!

With the uncertainty about causality how should we proceed? It is hard for even the most objective scientists to state his or her scientific opinion independently of his or her view on the public policy implications—and they rarely do so. If it were cheap to reduce particulate levels, most scientists would agree that it would be best to do so, and would state that the evidence is adequate to proceed from the statistical association between air pollution and health to the assignment of causality. The $60 billion per year would probably be worthwhile to save 15 thousand lives a year, but it would all be wasted if there is no health hazard at ambient 1996 levels, or if the hazard is due to some other cause. This makes politicians hesitate, and scientists to be hesitant about claiming a causal relationship.

Possible Actions for the U.S.

We divide the possible actions into three categories:

(1) additions to technology,

(2) modification of technology, and

(3) changing one technology for another.

Item (1): the societal actions of the last decade have been mostly concerned with minor additions to existing technology. These include:

(a) Improvement in end-use efficiency throughout all sectors of the economy. This is perhaps the most important step. There are many steps that can still be taken to improve end use efficiency *and save money*. The pay back for such actions is often of the order of years rather than the ten years of many investments. Included in this category might be wise use of solar heating to reduce energy demand.

(b) Sulfur removal at the chimney stack.

(c) Use of low sulfur fuels.

(d) Extensive washing of coal to remove the sulfur. As shown by the emissions estimates in Table 3.3, there are still considerable sulfur emissions in the U.S.

(e) Particulate suppression at the chimney stack. As shown in Table 3.3 the total particle emission is now reasonably low but this suppression must go beyond mere removal of most of the particulates by weight, and address the much harder task of removal of most of the fine particulates.

(f) Increase of efficiency of use of the power stations. This can reduce the amount of burning that is needed. It should be noted that the additions of (a), (c) and (d) to technology listed above, *reduce* power station efficiency, although they do reduce total particulate emissions.

(g) Use of natural gas to replace oil and coal now that it appears more plentiful. This accomplishes all of (a) through (f) above, although nitrogen oxide emissions must still be reduced.

(h) Increased nitrogen oxide and particle control for mobile sources (automobiles and trucks).

The second category (2) mostly applies to coal burning rather than to burning of the other fossil fuels:

(a) Gasification of coal and subsequent burning of the coal gas. It appears likely that gasification of coal can be accomplished without much particulate emission, and the burning of coal gas can be controlled more easily than the burning of coal itself, with less nitrogen oxide emissions. This then is similar to 1 (h) above.

(b) Accelerate the utilization of fluidized bed combustion.

Many of the procedures in the first two categories are already being implemented, but the reduction in the total of primary and secondary particulate emissions that is anticipated is closer to a factor of two than to the factor of one hundred needed to bring the risk down closer to the risks of other matters of EPA and public concern. This fact suggests urgent consideration of the replacement of technologies—the third category (3) above. This is replacing fossil fuel burning by some alternate source of energy supply. Most of these produce electricity as the end result, which can be adapted to most of the needs of society. These might include:

- replacement of inefficient technologies by fuel efficient technologies, using updated building, community and urban planning, telecommunications and appliance standards;

- hydropower;

- wind power, geothermal power and various solar power procedures;

- nuclear fission power; and

- nuclear fusion power (if ever it becomes practicable).

It should be obvious that integration of policies to improve public health by reducing air pollution should be integrated with global CO_2 reductions, strategies and energy security matters.

Replacement could be done even if such replacement would not be cost effective if the costs of air pollution are not taken into account. It could also be done in anticipation of future cost reductions in the technology. It seems likely that no one of these sources of replacement power will be applicable in all situations so that all must be considered.

International and Other Topical Issues

For an isolated island, such as New Zealand, simple calculations show that even quite large emissions of pollutants will not lead to large concentrations provided that tall chimney stacks are used. The pollution will blow out to sea and cover many thousands of miles before another landfall where the pollution can produce its adverse effects. This argument used to dominate governmental thinking in Great Britain, but the island is less isolated than formerly, and as a part of Europe has to consider pollution control in a more regional manner.

In the first edition of this book (Wilson et al. 1980) there was considerable discussion of transboundary pollution problems, and the legal resources and precedents that a jurisdiction might muster to persuade distant states or countries to control their emissions. This is now perceived as far less of a problem than formerly, as there is considerable cooperation among industrial countries. Table 10.1 gives a list of standards set by countries so far, and proposals in the U.S., to regulate particulate pollution.

In poor countries the Willingness to Pay will certainly be lower than in the U.S. The Willingness to Pay may be dominated by a Willingness to Please important trading partners. That this willingness to please is limited is clear from the international discussions with China on Global Climate Change. The Chinese feel no duty to reduce CO_2 emissions till

TABLE 10.1

Air Quality Standards for Particulate Matter

Agency	Standard	Comments
Japanese government	150 µg/m³	Indoor air standard for office buildings ($PM_{3.5}$)
US EPA	150 µg/m³	Outdoor National Ambient Air Quality Standard (PM_{10}, 24-hour average)
US EPA	50 µg/m³	Average annual ambient standard (PM_{10})
California	50 µg/m³	24-hour average (PM_{10})
California	30 µg/m³	Annual geometric mean(PM_{10})
US EPA Proposed	25–85 µg/m³	24-hour average ($PM_{2.5}$)
US EPA Proposed	15–30 µg/m³	Average annual ($PM_{2.5}$)
NRDC Proposed (Shprentz, 1966)	33 µg/m³	24-hour average (PM_{10})
NRDC Proposed	17 µg/m³	Average annual (PM_{10})
NRDC Proposed	20 µg/m³	24-hour average ($PM_{2.5}$)
NRDC Proposed	10 µg/m³	Average annual ($PM_{2.5}$)
WHO	120 µg/m³	European ambient air quality guideline, 24-hour total suspended particulates
WHO	70 µg/m³	European ambient air quality guideline, 24-hour thoracic particles (PM_{10})
German government	480 µg/m³	Outdoor standard, 1-hour total particulate concentration
Canadian government	40 µg/m³	Long-term indoor exposure guideline ($PM_{2.5}$)
Canadian government	150 µg/m³	One-hour indoor exposure guideline ($PM_{2.5}$)
ACGIH	10,000 µg/m³	Eight-hour PM_{10} occupational exposure guideline
OSHA	15,000 µg/m³	Occupational exposure guideline for total dust, not otherwise classified
OSHA	5,000 µg/m³	Occupational exposure guideline for respirable fraction, not otherwise classified
ASHRAE	50 µg/m³	Indoor exposure guideline, average annual (PM_{10})
ASHRAE	150 µg/m³	Indoor exposure guideline, 24-hour average (PM_{10})

their emissions *per capita* approach those of the U.S. It will require more than an improvement in public health to persuade developing countries to be concerned about air pollution.

The laws and regulations in the United States, and indeed many other jurisdictions, imply that there is a threshold below which there is no adverse effect on health at all. The U.S. Congress has demanded standards that achieve an adequate margin of safety, and thus must be below any scientifically determined threshold. Table 10.1 shows a list of such standards and some proposed changes.

The evidence in this book suggests that such a threshold may not exist, and certainly has not been determined. Therefore the U.S. and other countries must reexamine the legislative basis and perhaps consider a cost-benefit calculus for setting particulate air pollution standards.

A detailed discussion of the pros and cons of all these possible actions, national and international, is outside the chosen scope of this book.

Finale

We suggest what is often called a "no regrets" policy. That is to decide on energy systems with a small bias in favor of those energy technologies and strategies that reduce emissions of particulates or their precursors. To reduce risk, exposures must be reduced. Therefore regulatory strategies based on emissions, should be augmented by strategies based upon exposure reduction as the overarching principle of interest. These strategies can include pollution permitting and trading, public suasion through disclosure, a carbon tax, or even community-industry covenants. The principle must be to create new incentives for reducing the risk posed by air pollution that now is most likely to be directly proportional to the population exposure.

We also emphasize that the money spent on research in an attempt to understand the problem, while it seems large compared to some other research budgets, is small compared with the sum of money spent on emission reduction, or on the out-of-pocket costs of medical interventions.

In conclusion, we state our view that it is an international disgrace that although we have been burning coal and other fossil fuels for 800 years, we still do not burn them cleanly and we are not sure, in detail, of the effects of burning them dirtily.

Abbreviations

ACGIH	American Conference of Governmental Industrial Hygienists
AQCR	Air Quality Control Region
ASHRAE	American Society of Heating, Refrigerating, and Air-Conditioning Engineers
BACT	best available control technology
B α P	benzo (α) pyrene
BAL	brancheoalveolar lavage
$CaCO_3$	calcium carbonate
CAMP	Continuous Air Monitoring Project
CaO	calcium oxide
$(CH_3)_2S$	dimethyl sulfide
CO	carbon monoxide
CO_2	carbon dioxide
COH	coefficient of haze
COPD	chronic obstructive pulmonary (lung) disease
DL_{CO}	diffusing capacity of carbon monoxide
EC 50	effective concentration at which 50% of animals are affected
EPA	Environmental Protection Agency (U.S.)
ESP	electrostatic precipitator
ET	extrathoracic region of respiratory tract
ETS	environmental tobacco smoke
FEV	forced expiratory volume (a measure of lung function)
GEMS	Global Environmental Monitoring System
HEADS	Harvard/EPA Annular Denuder Sampler
H_2S	hydrogen sulfide
H_2SO_4	sulfuric acid
Hcl	hydrochloric acid
ICRP	International Commission on Radiological Protection
LDH	lactic dehydrogenase
LOLE	Loss of Life Expectancy
Mwe	megawatts electric
NAAQS	national ambient air quality standards (U.S.)

NADB	National Aerometric Data Bank
NAMS	National Air Monitoring System
NASN	National Air Surveillance Network (EPA)
$Na_2S_2O_5$	sodium metabisulfite
NaOH	sodium hydroxide
Na_2CO_3	sodium carbonate
NHANES	National Health and Nutrition Examination Surveys
NH_4HSO_4	ammonium bisulfate
NH_4OH	ammonium hydroxide
$(NH_4)_2SO_4$	ammonium sulfate
NLIN	non-linear estimation technique
NO_2	nitrogen dioxide
NO_x	nitrogen oxides
O_3	ozone
OH	hydroxyl radical
OSHA	Occupational Safety and Health Administration (U.S.)
PAH	polycyclic aromatic hydrocarbons
PAQS	primary air quality standard
PC	phagocytic capacity
POM	particulate organic matter
ppm	parts per million
PM	particulate matter
PSD	prevention of significant deterioration
rem	roentgen-equivalent-man
ROFA	residual oil fly ash
SAM	stationary ambient monitor
SIM	stationary indoor monitor
SLAMS	State and Local Air Monitoring Station
SMR	standard mortality ratio
SMS	Synchronous Meterorological Satellite
SMSA	standard metropolitan statistical area
SO_2	sulfur dioxide
SO_x	sulfur oxides
TBA	thio barbitonic acid
TB	tracheobronchial region of respiratory tract
TEOM	tapered element oscillating microbalance
TiO_2	titanium dioxide
TLC	total lung capacity
TSP	total suspended particles
VC	vital capacity
WHO	World Health Organization
WLW/BW	wet lung weight to body weight (ratio)
WMO	World Meterological Organization
$Zn(NH_4)_2(SO_4)_2$	ammonium sulfate

Glossary

acute (disease or effect): An immediate response with a short and generally severe course (often due to high pollutant concentrations for a short time (cf. *chronic*).

aerodynamic diameter: the diameter of a spherical particle that would fall at the same rate as the particle being discussed.

aerosol: a suspension of fine liquid or solid particles in a gas (usually air).

ambient level: the level of pollutant in the general environment.

antagonism: where the combined action of two or more pollutants is less that the sum of the actions of each acting separately (cf. *synergism*).

anthropogenic: of human origin.

asphyxiation: the action of suffocation by depriving tissue of oxygen.

bronchitis: inflammation of the bronchial tubes.

bronchoconstriction: reduced size of the bronchial tubes by contraction of the bronchial walls.

bronchodilators: usually a chemical spray used by asthmatics and others to dilate the bronchi.

carcinogenic: cancer causing.

chronic: a disease response that lingers a long time and arises slowly, usually due to exposure to continuous, low concentrations of pollutants (cf. *acute*).

combustion: the process of burning.

cyclone: a device to separate particles using a rotating vortex as in a cyclone.

diffusion capacity: the abilty of a material to diffuse into a surface (for example of the lung).

dose-response: the relationship between the dose to which a person (organism) is exposed and the response to that dose. Most responses increase monotonically with dose.

edema: a swelling due to effusion of watery fluid into intercellular spaces.

epidemiology: the study of epidemics of human disease by observation of the human populations.

fly-ash: small solid ash particles from the noncombustible portion of fuel that are small enough to escape with the exhaust gases.

Gaussian model (distribution): a Gaussian distribution was derived by Karl Friedrich Gauss, a famous 19th century scientist as a normal (standard) distribution. It is expressed by:

$$P(x)dx = \frac{1}{\sigma\sqrt{2\pi}} \exp\frac{(x - \bar{x})^2}{2\sigma^2} dx$$

where: *P(x)* is the probability of finding the value of a quantity between *x* and *x + dx*.
σ is called the *Standard Deviation*.
χ is called the *Mean*.

harvesting: the sudden death or disease of people who have been rendered sensitive by previous disease (or previous exposures).

haze: obscuration of the earth's atmosphere usually over large areas.

homeostasis: a tendency toward stability of the body.

hyperplazia: abnormal multiplication of the normal cells in tissue.

hypertrophy: excessive enlargement of a part or an organ.

inertial impactor: a device to separate particles by their different inertial impact.

inhalable particles: those particles that are breathed in and reach the respiratory tract.

inhalable particles (EPA definition): particles with aerodynamic diameters less than 10 μg (PM_{10}).

in vivo: within living organisms.

in vitro: outside of living organisms (lit. *in glass*).

lung: *alveoli*—small sacs through which gas exchange takes place.
bronchi—branching air passages in the lung.
bronchioli—final branching of the bronchi.
cilia—small hairlike processes that move mucus in the bronchi.
epithelium—the lining walls of the lung.
macrophage—a wandering cell that ingests (phagocytizes) foreign particles.

measurements:

length: 1 kilometer (km) = 1,000 meters (m) = 10^5 cm = 10^6 mm = 10^9 μm.

weight: 1 metric tonne = 1,000 kilograms (kg) = 1 million (10^6) grams (g) = 10^9 milligrams (mg) = 10^{12} micrograms (μg) = 10^{15} nanograms (ng).

1 part per million (ppm) of a pollutant in water is usually 1 gram weight of the pollutant for every million grams (1,000 kg) of water.

1 part per million (ppm) of a pollutant in air is usually 1 cc of pollutant volume per million cc (1000 liters) of air. Then 1 ppm in air = (Molecular weight/24.45) mg/m^3.

1 μg/m^3 is 1 microgram in a cubic meter.

meteorology: a study of the weather and processes in the atmosphere.

potentiation: where a pollutant that produces no response increases the response to another pollutant.

proportional: two quantities are proportional to each other when if one doubles in size the other does also. if a human disease incidence doubles in response to doubling of a pollutant, it is said to be proportional.

morbidity: sickness.

mortality: death.

necrosis: death of tissue.

particles: small objects, usually solid but sometimes liquid, that can be carried (suspended) by the air. They come in different sizes. In this book we distinguish Total Suspended Particles and particles of sizes less than 2.5 or 10 um in diameter ($PM_{2.5}$ and PM_{10} respectively).

plume: the cloud of steam or smoke (or sometimes invisible cloud) that comes from a chimney stack (or other source) and blows downwind.

point source: a source of pollutant that is in one specific location such as a chimney stack.

pollutant: any material entering the environment that has undesired effects.

respirable particles: see inhalable particles.

sampler:
>*dichotomous*—a particle capture device that separates particles into two size categories (e.g < 2 μm, > 2μm).
>*high volume*—a particle capture device that samples all suspended aerosols or TSP.

sedimentation: gravitational settling.

sink: a place where pollutants get absorbed or just "disappear" e.g. the sea.

sorbed: present on surface of particles.

source: a place where pollutants are emitted—for example a chimney stack or automobile exhaust pipe.

Stokes' law: the law enunciated by the 19th century mathematician and physicist Stokes that governs the fall of small particles through a fluid.

synergism: a situation where the combined action of two or more pollutants is greater than the sum of the actions of each acting separately (cf. *antagonism*).

threshold: a pollutant concentration below which no deleterious (adverse) effects occur.

trace: a very small amount of a material.

tonne: a metric ton which is 1,000 kilograms (cf. *measurements*).

topography: the detailed description and delineation of the geographical features of a locality.

toxicology: the study of toxic materials and the way in which they interact with animals including people.

References

Abbey, D.E., Mills, P.K., and Beeson, W.L. (1991) "Long-Term Ambient Concentrations of Total Suspended Particulates and Oxidants as Related to Incidence of Chronic Disease in California Seventh-Day Adventists" *Environ. Health Perspect.* 94:43–50.

Abbey, D.E., Petersen, F., Mills, P.K., and Beeson, W.L. (1993) "Long-Term Ambient Concentrations of Total Suspended Particulates, Ozone, and Sulfur Dioxide and Respiratory Symptoms in a Non-Smoking Population" *Arch. Environ. Health.* 48:33–46.

Ackland, G.G., Hartwell, T.D., Johnson, T.R., and Whitemore, R.W. (1985) "Measuring Human Exposure to Carbon Monoxide in Washington, D.C. and Denver, Colorado, During the Winter 1982–1983" *Environ. Sci. and Tech.* 19:911–918.

Adams, W.C. (1993) "Measurement of Breathing Rate and Volume in Routinely Performed Daily Activities." Davis, CA: University of California, Physical Education Department, Human Performance Laboratory: contract no. A033–205.

Ahlberg, M.S., and Winchester, J.W. (1978) "Dependence of aerosol sulfur particle size on relative humidity" *Atmos. Environ.* 12:1631–1632.

Alarie, Y.C., Krumm, A.A., Busey, W.M., et al. (1972) "Long-term Exposure to Sulfuric Dioxide in Cynomolgus Monkeys" *Arch. Environ. Health* 24:115.

Alarie, Y.C., Krumm. A.A., Busey, W.M. et al. (1975) "Long-term Exposure to Sulfur Dioxide, Sulfuric Acid Mist and Their Mixtures" *Arch. Environ. Health* 30:254.

Amdur, M.O., Schultz, R.Z. and Drinker, P. (1952) "Toxicity of Sulfuric Acid Mist to Guinea Pigs" *Arch. Ind. Hyg. Occup. Med.* 5·1.

Amdur, M.O. and Drinker, P. (1954) "Effect of Combination of SO_2 and H_2SO_4, on Human Subjects" Presented at the American Industrial Hygiene Association Meeting, Chicago, IL, May.

Amdur, M.O. and Corn, M. (1963) "The Irritant Potency of Zinc Ammonium Sulfate of Different Particle Sizes" *Amer. Ind. Hyg. Assoc. J.* 24:326.

Amdur, M.O.(1964) "The Effects of High Flow-Resistance on the Response of Guinea Pigs to Irritants" *Amer. Ind. Hyg. Assoc. J.* 25:564.

Amdur, M.O. (1970) "The Impact of Air Pollutants on Physiologic Responses of the Respiratory Tract" *Philosophic Soc.* 114:3.

Amdur, M.O. (1974) "The Long Road from Donora: 1974 Cummings Memorial Lecture" *Amer. Ind. Hyg. Assoc. J.* 35:589.

Amdur, M.O., Dubriel, M. and Creasia, D.A. (1978) "Respiratory Response Guinea Pigs to Low Levels of Sulfuric Acid" *Environ. Res.* 15:418.

Amdur, M.O., McCarthy, J.F. and Gill, M.W. (1983) "Effect of Mixing Conditions on Irritant Potency of Zinc Oxide and Sulfur Dioxide" *Amer. Indust. Hyg. Assoc. J.* 44:7.

Amdur, M.O., Sarofim, A.F., Neville, M. et al. (1986) "Coal Combustion Aerosols and SO_2: An Interdisciplinary Analysis "*Environ. Sci. Technol.* 20:138.

Amdur, M.O., Chen, I.C., Guty, J. et al. (1988) "Speciation and Pulmonary Effects of Acid SO_2 Formed on Surface of Ultrafine Zinc Oxide Aerosols" *Atmos. Environ.* 22:557.

Amdur, M.O. (1989) "Sulfuric Acid: The Animals Tried to Tell Us" in the 1989 Herbert E. Stokinger Lecture, *Appl. Ind. Hyg.* 4(8):189–197.

Amdur, M.O. and Chen, I.C. (1989) "Furnace-Generated Acid Aerosols: Speciation and Pulmonary Effects" *Environ. Health Perspec.* 79:147–150.

American Lung Association (1993) "Breath in Danger II: Estimation of Populations-at-Risk of Adverse Health Consequences in Areas Not in Attainment with National Ambient Air Quality Standards of the Clean Air Act" *American Lung Association* Washington, D.C.

Anderson, K.R. and Avol, E.L. (1988) "Controlled exposures of volunteers to respirable carbon and sulfuric acid aerosols" *J. Air Waste Manage. Assoc.* 42:770–6.

Anderson, P.J. and Wilson, J.D. (1990) "Respiratory tract deposition of ultrafine particles in subjects with obstructive or restrictive lung disease" *Chest* 97:1115–20.

Appel, B.R., Povard, V., and Kothny, E.L. (1988) "Loss of nitric acid within inlet devices for atmospheric sampling" *Atmos. Environ.* 22:2535–2540.

Appel, B.R., Tokiwa, Y., Haik, M., and Kothny E.L. (1984) "Artifact particulate sulfate, and nitrate formation on filter media" *Atmos. Environ.* 18:409.

Appel, B. R., Povard, V., and Kohny, E. L. (1988) "Loss of nitric acid within inlet devices intended to exclude coarse particles during atmospheric sampling" *Atmos. Environ.* 11:2535–2540.

Archer, V.E. (1990) "Air pollution and fatal lung disease in three Utah counties" *Arch. Environ. Health* 45:325–334.

Armytage, W.H. (1961) "A Social History of Engineering" *MIT Press.* Cambridge, Massachusetts.

Bahadori, T., Suh, H., and Koutrakis, P. (1996) "Personal, Indoor, and Outdoor Concentrations of PM_{10} and $PM_{2.5}$ for 10 COPD Patients Living at Home" Presented at *2nd Colloquium on Particulate Air Pollution and Health.* Park City, Utah, May 1–3, 1996.

Bailey, M.R. and Fry, F.A. (1982) "The long-term clearance kinetics of insoluble particles from the human lung" *Ann. Occup. Hyg.* 26:273–90.

Bascom, R, et al. (1996) "Health Effects of Outdoor Air Pollution" *Amer. J. Crit. Care Med.* 153:3–50.

Bates, D.V. and Sizto, R. (1987) "Air pollution and hospital admissions in southern Ontario: the acid summer haze effect" *Environ. Research* 43:317–331.

Bates, D.V. (1989) *Respiratory function in disease,* 3rd ed. Philadelphia: W.B. Saunders.

Bates, D.V. (1980) "The health effects of air pollution" *J. Resp. Disease* 1:29–37.

Bates, D.V. and Sizto, R. (1989) "The Ontario Air Pollution Study: Identification of the Causative Agent" *Environ. Health Perspect.* 79:69–72.

Bates, D.V. (1992) "Health Indices of the Adverse Effects of Air Pollution: the Question of Coherence" *Environ. Research.* 59:336–49.

Bates, D.V. (1995) Commentary on Colloquium on Particulate Pollution and Human Mortality and Morbidity" *Inhal. Toxicol.* 7(1):iv–viii.

Bates, D.V., Baker-Anderson, M., and Sizto, R. (1990) "Asthma attack periodicity: A study of hospital emergency visits in Vancouver" *Environ. Research* 51:51–70.

Beaty, T.H., Newill, C.A., Cohen, B.H., Tockman, M.S., Bryant, S.H., and Spurgeon, H.A. (1985) "Effects of pulmonary function on mortality" *J. Chronic Disease* 38:703–710.

Beaver H. (Chairman) (1953) "Interim report" (on London air pollution incident) *Committee on Air Pollution: Cmd 9011,* Her Majesty's Stationary Office, London.

Biersteker, K., H. de Graaf, and Ch. A. G. Nass, (1965) "Indoor Air Pollution in Rotterdam Homes," *Int. J. Air Water Poll.* 9:343.

Biggins, P. and Harrison, R.M. (1979) "Atmospheric chemistry of automotive lead" *Environ. Sci. and Technol.* 13:558–564.

Biswas, P., Jones, C.L., and Flagan, R.C. (1987) "Distortion of size distributions by condensation and evaporation in aerosol instruments" *Aerosol Sci. and Technol.* 7:231–246.

Blair, A., Burg, J., Foran, J., Gibb, H., Greenland, S., Morris, R., Raabe, G., Savitz, D., Teta, J., Wartenberg, D., Wong, O., and Zimmerman, R., (1995) "Guidelines for Application of Meta-Analysis in Environmental Epidemiology" *Regul. Toxicol. Pharmacol.* 22:189–197.

Bobak, B. and Leon, D.A. (1992) "Air pollution and infant mortality in the Czech Republic" 1986–1988. *Lancet* 340:1010–1014.

Brain, J.D., and Valdberg, P.A. (1979) "Deposition of aerosols in respiratory tract" *Amer. Rev. Resp. Disease* 120:1325.

Braman, R.S., Shelley, T.J., and McClenney, W.A. (1982) "Tungstic acid for the preconcentration and determination of gaseous and particulate ammonia and nitric acid in ambient air" *Analytical Chem.* 54:356–364, 1982.

Brauer, M., P. Koutrakis and J. D. Spengler, (1989) "Personal Exposures to Acidic Aerosols and Gases" *Environ. Sci. Technol.,* 23:1408.

Braun-Fahlander, C., Ackermann-Leibrich, U., Schwartz, J., and Gnehm, H.P., Rutishauser, M., and Wanner, H.U. (1992) "Air pollution and respiratory symptoms in preschool children" *Amer. Rev. Resp. Disease.* 145:42–47.

Brimblecombe P. (1987) "The Big Smoke" *Routledge, Chapman & Hall,* London, England.

Brosset, C., Andreasson, K., and Ferm, M. (1975) "The nature and possible origin of acid particles observed at the Swedish west coast" *Atmos. Environ.* 9:631–642.

Brunekreef, B., Kinney, P.L., Ware, J.H., Dockery, D., Speizer, F.E., Spengler, J.D., and Ferris, B.G. (1991) "Sensitive subgroups and normal variation in pulmonary function response to air pollution episodes" *Environ. Health Perspect.* 90:189–193.

Buat-Menard, P. (1979) "Influence de la retombée atmospherique sur la chimie des metaux en trace dans la matière en suspension de l' Atlantique Nord" *Ph.D. Dissertation, University of Paris.*

Bucher, A., and Lucas, C. (1983) "Retombees estivales des poussieres sahariennes sur l'Europe" *Rev. de Geologie Dynamique et de Geographie Physique* 24:153–165.

Burge, H.A., Otten, J. and Chatigny, M. (1987) "Guidelines for assessment and sampling of saprophytic bioaerosols in indoor environment" *Appl. Ind. Hyg.* 2(5):1–10.

Burge, H.A., and Solomon, W.R. (1987) "Sampling and analysis of biological aerosols" *Atmos. Environ.* 21:45.

Burnett, R.T., Dales, R.E., Raizenne, M.E., Krewski, D., Summers, P.W., Roberts, G.R., Raad-Young, M., Dann, T., and Brook, J. (1994) "Effects of low ambient levels of ozone and sulfates on the frequency of respiratory admissions to Ontario hospitals" *Environ. Research* 65:172–194.

Burnett, R.T., Dales, R.E., Krewski, D., et al. (1995) "Associations Beween Ambient Particulate Sulfate and Admissions to Ontario Hospitals for Cardiac and respiratory Diseases" *Amer. J.Epidemiology* in press.

Burton, R.M., Suh, H.H., and Koutrakis, P. (1996) "Spatial Variation in Particulate Concentrations within Metropolitan Philadelphia" *Environ. Sci. and Tech.* 30(2): 400–407.

Cadle, S.H., Groblicki, P.J., and Mulawa, P.A. (1993) "Problems in the sampling and analysis of carbon particulate" *Atmos. Environ.* 17:593.

Camilli A.E., Burrows B., Knudson R.J., et al. (1987) "Longitudinal changes in FEV_1 in adults: Methodologic considerations and findings in healthy non-smokers" *Amer. Rev. Respir. Disease* 135:794–9.

Chambers, L.A. (1977) "Classification and extent of problems" In *Air Pollution*, A. Stern, ed. New York, Academic Press.

Chan, T., and Lippmann, M. (1977) "Particle collection efficiencies of air sampling cyclones: an empirical theory" *Environ. Sci. and Technol.* 11:377.

Chappie, M. and Lave, L., (1982) "The health effects of air pollution: a reanalysis" *J. Urban Economics* 12:346–76.

Chatigny, M.A., Macher, J.M., Burge, H.A., and Solomon, W.R. (1989) "Sampling airborne microorganisms and aeroallergens" In *Air Sampling Instruments*, edited by S.V. Hering. American Conference of Governmental Industrial Hygienists, Inc., Cincinnati, OH, 1989.

Chen, L.C., Fine J.M., Qu Q.S., et al. (1992) "Effects of fine and ultrafine sulrfuric acid aerosols in guinea pigs: alterations in alveolar macrophage function and intracellular pH" *Toxicol. Appl. Pharmacol.* 113:109–17.

Chen, L.C., Lam, H.F., Ainsworth, D., Guty, J., and Amdur, M.O. (1987) "Functional Changes in the Lungs of Guinea Pigs Exposed to Sodium Sulfite Aerosols" *Toxicol. Appl. Pharmacol.* 89:1.

Chen, L.C., Miller, P.D. , Lam, H.F., Guty, J., and Amdur, M.O. (1991) "Sulfuric Acid-Layered Ultrafine Particles Potentiate Ozone-Induced Airway Injury" *J. Toxicol. Environ. Health* 34:337.

Chestnut, L.G., Schwartz, J., Savitz, D.A., and Burchfiel, C.M. (1991) "Pulmonary Function and Ambient Particulate Matter: Epidemiological Evidence from NHANES I" *Arch. Environ. Health* 46:135–144.

Christensen J. H. and Berkowicz R. (1991) "Modelling Photochemical Pollution by an Eulerian Long-Range Transport Model" in *Air pollution Modelling and its Application,* vol VIII (ed: van Dop H. and Steyn D.G.) Plenum Press, New York.

Ciocco, A., and Thompson, D.J. (1961) "A follow-up on Donora ten years after: methodology and findings" *Amer. J. Public Health* 51:155–164.

Clarke, A.J., D.H. Lucas, and F.F. Ross. (1970) "Tall stacks: how effective are they?" *Second International Air Pollution Conference,* Washington, D.C.

Cochran, W.G. (1970) "Some Effects of Errors of Measurement on Multiple Correlation" *J. Amer. Stat. Assoc.* 65:22–34.

Cohen, D., Arai, S.F.and Brain J.D. (1979) "Smoking Impairs Long-term Clearance from the Lung" *Science* 204:514–517.

Commins, B.T. and Waller, R.E. (1967) "Observation from a Ten-year Study at a Site in the City of London" *Atmos. Environ.* 1:49.

Corn, M., (1976) "Properties of Nonviable Particles in Air," in *Air Pollution,* A.C. Stern, Ed., 3rd Ed. I(3):77, Academic Press, New York.

Costa, D.L., Lehmann, J.R., Frazier, L.T., Doerfler, D., and Giho, A. (1995) "Pulmonary Hypertension: A Possible Risk Factor in Particulate Toxicity" *Amer. J. Respir. Crit. Care Med.* 151:A840.

Craig, N.L., Marker, A.B.and Novakov, T. (1974) "Determination of the Chemical States of Sulfur in Ambient Pollutant Aerosols by X-ray Photoelectron Spectroscopy" *Atmos. Environ.* 8:15.

Cronn, D.R., Charlson, R.J., Knights, R.L., Crittenden, A.L., and Appel, B.R. (1977) "A survey of the molecular nature of primary and secondary components of particles in urban air by high-resolution mass spectrometry" *Atmos. Environ.* 11:929.

Courtney, W.J., Shaw, R.W., and Dzubay, T.G. (1982) "Precision and accuracy of a b-gauge for aerosol mass determination" *Environ. Sci. and Technol.* 16:236–239.

Coutant R.W., Callahan P.J., Kuhlman M.R., and Lewis R.G. (1989) "Design and performance of a high-volume compound annular denuder" *Atmos. Environ.* 23(10):2205–2211.

Crawford, M. and Wilson, R., (1996) "Low Dose Linearity: The Rule or the Exception?" *Human and Ecological Risk Assessment* 2(2):305–330.

Dasgupta, P.K., De Cesare, K.B., and Brummer, M. (1982) "Determination of S(IV) in Particulate Matter" *Atmos. Environ.* 16:917.

Dassen, W., Brunekreef, B., Hoek, G., Hofschreuder, P., Staatsen, B., de Groot, H., Schouten, E. and Bierstekor, K., (1986) "Decline in children's in children's pulmonary function during an air pollution episode" *J. Air Poll. Control Assoc.* 36:1223–1227.

Davidson, R.L., Natusch, D.F.S., Wallace, J.R., and Evans, C.A., (1974) "Trace Elements in Fly Ash. Dependence of Concentration on Particle Size" *Environ. Sci. Technol.* 8:1107.

Department of Health and Human Services (DHHS) (1991) "Guidelines for the Diagnosis and Management of Asthma" *National Asthma Education Program Expert Panel Report. Publication No. 91–3042.* Bethesda, MD: U.S. Government Printing Office.

Der Simonian R., and Laird, N.M. (1986) "Meta-Analysis in Clinical Trials" in *Controlled Clinical Trials* 7:177–178.

Dirgo, J. and Leith, D. (1985) "Cyclone collection efficiency: comparison of experimental results with theoretical predictions" *Aerosol Sci. and Technol.* 4:401.

Dockery, D.W. and Pope, C.A., III (1994) "Acute respiratory effects of particulate air pollution" *Ann. Rev. Public Health* 15:107–132.

Dockery, D.W., Speizer, F.E., Ferris, B.G. Jr., Ware, J.H., Louis, T.A. and Spiro, A. III (1988) "Cumulative and reversible effects of lifetime smoking on simple tests of lung function in adults" *Amer. Rev. Respir. Disease* 137:286–292.

Dockery, D.W., Pope, C.A. III, Xu, X., Spengler, J.D., Ware, J.H., Ray, M.E., Ferris, B.G. Jr., and Speizer, F.E. (1993) "An association between air pollution and mortality in six U.S. cities" *New England J. Med.* 329:1753–1759.

Dockery, D. W., and Spengler, J. D. (1981a) "Indoor-Outdoor Relationships of Sulfates and Particles" *Atmos. Environ.* 15:335–343.

Dockery, D. W. and J. D. Spengler, (1981b) "Personal Exposure to Respirable Particulates and Sulfates," *J. Air Poll. Control Assoc.* 31:153–159.

Dockery, D.W., Ware, J.H., Ferris, B.G., Jr., Speizer, F.E., Cook, N.R., and Herman, S.M. (1982) "Change in pulmonary function in children associated with air pollution episodes" *J. Air Poll. Control Assoc.* 32:937–942.

Dockery, D.W., Schwartz, J., and Spengler, J.D. (1992) "Air pollution and daily mortality: Associations with particulates and acid aerosols" *Environ. Research* 59:362–373.

Dockery, D.W., Speizer, F.E., Stram, D.O., Ware, J.H., Spengler, J.D., and Ferris, B.G. Jr. (1989) "Effects of inhalable particles on respiratory health of children" *Amer. Rev. Resp. Disease* 139:587–594.

Dockery, D.W., Schwartz, J., and Spengler, J.D. (1992) "Air pollution and daily mortality: Associations with particulates and acid aerosols" *Environ. Research* 59:362–373.

Dockery, D.W., Pope, C.A. III, Xu, X., Spengler, J.D., Ware, J.H., Fay, M.E., Ferris, B.G., and Speizer, F.E. (1993a) "Mortality risks of air pollution: a prospective cohort study" *New England J.Medicine* 329:1753–1759.

Dockery, D.W., Damokash, A.I., Neas, L.M. Raizenne, M., Spengler, J.D., Koutrakis, P., Ware, J.H., and Speizer, F.E. (1993b) "Health effects of acid aerosols on North American children: Respiratory symptoms and illness" Presented at the *American Lung Association/American Thoracic Society International Conference*, San Francisco, May 16–19.

Dockery, D.W. and Pope, C.A. III (1994) "Acute Respiratory Effects of Particulate Air Pollution" *Ann. Revs. Public Health* 15:107–132.

Dockery, D.W. and Pope, C.A. III (1996) To be published.

Doll R, and R. Peto, (1976) "Mortality in Relation to Smoking: 20 years of Observation on male British Doctors" *Brit. Med. J.* 2:1525–1536.

Dreher, K., Jaskot, R., Richards, J., Lehmann, J., Winsett, D., Hoffmann, A., Costa, D. (1990) "Acute Pulmonary Toxicity of Size-Fractionated Ambient Air Particulate Matter" Presented at the American Thoracic Society Conference, May 10–15, 1996, New Orleans, LA.

Dreher, K., Jaskot, R., Richards, J., Lehmann, J., Winsett, D., Hoffmann, A., Costa, D. (1996) "Acute Pulmonary Toxicity of Size-Fractionated Ambient Air Particulate Matter" *Amer. J. Respir. Crit. Care Med.* 153:A15.

Driscoll, K.E., Strzelecki, J., Hassenbein, D., Janssen, Y., Marsh, J., Öberd rster, G., Mossman, B.T. (1994) "Tumor Necrosis Factor (TNF): Evidence for the Role of TNF in Increased Expression of Manganese Superoxide Dismutase After Inhalation of Mineral Dusts" *Ann. Amer. J. Respir. Cell Mol. Biol.* 6:535.

Duan, N. (1982) "Models for Human Exposure to Air Pollution" *Environ. Int.* 8:305–309.

Durham, J.L., Wilson, W.E., and Bailey, E.B. (1978) "Application of an SO_2 denuder for continuous measurement of sulfur in submicrometric aerosols" *Atmos. Environ.* 12:883–886.

Dzubay, T. G. and R. K. Stevens, (1975) "Ambient Air Analysis with the Dichotomous Sampler and X-Ray Fluorescence Spectrometer," *Env. Sci. Technol.* 9(7):633.

Dzubay, T.G. (1984) "Recent advances in energy-dispersive XRF analysis of aerosol samples. *Atmos. Environ.*, 18:1555–1566.

Eatough, D.J and Hansen, L.D. (1980) "S(IV) Chemistry in Smelter Produced Particulate Matter" *Amer. J. Indust. Med.* 1:435.

Eatough, D.J., Richter, B.E., Eatough, N.L., and Hansen, L.D. (1981) "Sulfur Chemistry in Smelter and Power Plant Plumes in Western United States" *Atmos. Environ.* 15:2241.

Ellison, J.M., and Waller, R.E. (1978) "A review of sulphur oxides and particulate matter as air pollutants with particular reference to effects on health in the United Kingdom" *Environ. Research* 16:302–325.

Environmental Protection Agency (EPA) (1982) "Review of the National Ambient Air Quality Standards for Particulate Matter: Assessment of Scientific and Technical Information" Office of Air Quality Planning and Standards, U.S. EPA, North Carolina, EPA-450/5-82-001.

Environmental Protection Agency (EPA) (1986) "Industrial Source Complex (ISC) Dispersion Model User's Guide" 2nd Edition Vol 1 EPA-450/46-005a.

Environmental Protection Agency (EPA) (1989) "Health effects and aerometrics: an acid aerosols issue paper" Report no. 600/8–88-005F. Office of Health and Environmental Assessment, Washington, D.C. U.S. Government Printing Office.

Environmental Protection Agency (EPA) (1990) "Non-occupational pesticide exposure study (NOPES)," Final Report. EPA/600/3–90/003.

Environmental Protection Agency (EPA) (1993) "Natural Air Quality and Trends Reports-1992" EPA A54/R-93-031.

Environmental Protection Agency (EPA) (1995a) "EPA study of indoor air pollution."

Environmental Protection Agency (EPA) (1995b) "EPA Review of the National Ambient Air Quality Standards for Particulate Matter" *External Review draft* November.

Euler, G.L., Abbey, D.E., Magie, A.R., and Hodgkin, J.E. (1987) "Chronic obstructive pulmonary disease symptom effects of long-term cumulative exposure to ambient levels of total suspended particulates and sulfur dioxide in California Seventh-Day Adventist residents" *Arch. Environ. Health* 42:213–222.

Evans, J.S., Tosteson, T., and Kinney, P.L. (1984) "Cross-sectional mortality studies and air pollution risk assessment" *Environ. Int.* 10:55–83.

Evans, J.S., Özkaynak, H. and Wilson, R. (1982) "The use of models in public health risk analysis" *J. Energy & Environ.* 1:1–20.

Evans, J.S., Gray G.M., Sielken, R.L. Jr, Smith A.E., Valdez-Flores C., and Graham J.D., (1994a) "The use of Probabilistic Expert Judgement in Uncertainty Analysis of Carcinogenic Potency" *Regul. Toxicol. and Pharmacol.* 20:15–36.

Evans, J.S., Graham J.D., Gray G.M., and Sielken, R.L. Jr, (1994b) "A Distributional Approach to Characterizing Low-Dose Cancer Risk" *Risk Analysis* 14:25–35.

Evelyn, J. (1661) "Fumigorum or the Inconvenience of the Aer and Smoake of London Dissipated: Together with some remdies humbly proposed" 2nd printing 1772 quoted in *Pitts and Metcalf 1969.*

Fairley D. (1990) "The relationship of daily mortality to suspended particulates in Santa Clara County, 1980–1986" *Environ. Health Perspect.* 89:159–68.

Fawal, H.A.N. and Schlesinger, R.B. (1994) "Nonspecific Airway Hyperresponsiveness Induced by Inhalation Exposure to Sulfuric Acid Aerosol: An *in Vitro* Assessment" *Toxicol. Appl. Pharm.* 125:70.

Ferm, M. (1979) "Method for determination of atmospheric ammonia" *Atmos. Environ.* 13:1385–1393.

Ferris, B.G. Jr., (1978) "Health Effects of Exposure to Low Levels of Regulated Air Pollutants: A Critical Review," *J. Air Poll. Control Assoc.* 28:482.

Ferris, B.G., Speizer, F.E., Spengler, J.D., Dockery, D.W., Bishop, Y.M.M., Wolfson, M., and Humble, C. (1979) "Effects of Sulfur Oxides and Respirable Particles on Human Health: Methodology and Demography of Population in Study," *Amer. Rev. Resp. Disease* 120:767–779.

Ferron G., Haider B., and Kreyling W.G. (1985) "A method for the approximation of the relative humidity in the upper human airways" *Bull. Math. Biol.* 47:565–89.

Findeisen, W. (1935) "Uber das Absetzen kleiner in der Luft suspendierten Teilchen in der menschlichen Lunge bei der Atmung" *Arch. Ges. Physiol.* 236:367.

Fine J.M., and Gordon T. (1987) "The role of titratable acidity in acid aerosol-induced bronchoconstriction" *Amer. Rev. Resp. Dis.* 146:626–32.

Finlayson-Pitts, B.J., and Pitts, J.N. (1986) "Atmospheric Chemistry" *John Wiley & Sons,* New York.

Firket, J. (1931) "The Cause of the Symptoms found in the Meuse Valley during the Fog of December 1930" *Bull. Roy. Acad. Med. Belgium* 11:683–741.

Firket J., (1936) "Fog along the Meuse Valley" *Trans. Faraday Soc.* 32:1107–1197.

First, M.W. (1989) "Air sampling and analysis for contaminants: an overview" In *Air Sampling Instruments*, edited by S.V. Hering. *American Conference of Governmental Industrial Hygienists, Inc.*, Cincinnati, OH.

Fisher, A., Chestnut, L.G., and Violette D.M. (1989) "The Value of Reducing Risks of Death: A Note on the New Evidence" *J. Policy Analysis and Manage.* 8(1):88–100.

Fitz, D.R. (1990) "Reduction of the positive artifact on quartz filters" *Aerosol Sci. and Technol.* 12:142–148.

Forrest, J., Spandau, D.J., Tanner, R.L., and Newman, L. (1982) *Atmos. Environ.* 16:1473–1485.

Frampton M.W., Voter K.Z., Morrow P.E, et al. (1992) "Sulfuric acid aerosol exposure in humans assessed by bronchoalveolar lavage" *Amer. Rev. Respir. Disease* 146:626–32.

Gavett, S.H., Madison, S.L., Winsett, D.W., McGee, J.K., and Costa, D.L. (1996) "Metal and Sulfate Composition of Residual Oil Fly Ash Determine Airway Hyperreactivity and Lung Injury in Sprague-Dawley Rats" *Amer. J. Respir. Crit. Care Med.* 153:A542.

Gearhart, J.M. and Schlesinger, R.B. (1989) "Sulfuric Acid-Induced Changes in the Physiology and Structure of the Tracheobronchial" *Environ. Health Perspect.* 79:127.

Gemmill, D.deJ., (1972) "Manchester in the Victorian Age: Factors Influencing the Design and Implementation of Smoke Abatement Policy," an Essay in Partial Fulfillment of a Masters Degree in Public Health, Yale University, New Haven, CT.

Ghio, A.J., Stonehuemer, J., Prichard, R.J. Piantadosi, C.A., Quigley, D.R., Dreher, K.L., and Costa, D.L. (1996) "Humic-Like Substances in Air Pollution Particulates Correlate with Concentrations of Transition Metals and Oxidant Generation" *Inhal. Toxicol.* (In press).

Godleski, J.J. Sioutas, C., Katler, M., Koutrakis, P. (1996) "Death from Inhalation of Concentrated Ambient Air Particles in Animal Models of Pulmonary Disease" *Amer. J. Respir. Crit. Care Med.* 153:A15.

Goldsmith, J. R. and L. T. Friberg, (1977) "Effects on Human Health," in *Air Pollution*, A.C. Stern, Ed., 3rd Ed., II(7):457, *Academic Press*, New York.

Gordian, M., S. Morris, H. Özkaynak, J. Xue and J. Spengler, (1995) "Health Effects of Particulate Pollution in Anchorage, Alaska," Presented at the *International Conference on Particulate Matter: Health and Regulatory Issues,* Pittsburgh, PA, April 4–6.

Gordon, G.E. (1984) "Considerations for design of source apportionment studies" *Atmos. Environ.* 18:1567–1582.

Gregor, J.J. (1976) "Mortality and air quality: the 1968–1972 Allegheny County Experience." Center for the Study of Environmental Policy, Pennsylvania State University, University Park, Pennsylvania.

Gudikesen, P.H., Sullivan, T.J. and Harvey, T.F (1986) "The Current State of ARAC and its application to the Chernobyl Event" *Lawrence Livermore National Laboratory report.* Livermore, CA, UCRL-95562.

Hansen, A.D.A., Rosen, H., and Novakov, T. (1984) "The aethalometer-an instrument for real-time measurement of optical absorption by aerosol particles" *Sci. Tot. Environ.* 36:191–196.

Hansen, A.D.A., and Rosen, H. (1990) "Individual measurements of the emission factor of aerosol black carbon in automobile plumes" *J. Air Waste Manag. Assoc.* 40:1654–1657.

Hayder et al. (1992) *Inhal. Toxicol.* 4(3) (five papers).

Hering S.V., Flagan R.C., and S.K. Friedlander. (1978) "Design and evaluation of a new low pressure impactor-1" *Environ. Sci. Technol.* 12:667–673.

Hering, S.V. (1989) "Inertial and gravitational collectors" In *Air Sampling Instruments* edited by S.V. Hering. American Conference of Governmental Industrial Hygienists, Inc., Cincinnati, OH.

Herington, C.F. (1920) "Powdered Coal as a Fuel," *Van Nostrand-Reinhold*, Princeton, NJ.

Hill, A.B (1965) "The Environment and Disease: Association and Causation?" in *Proc. Roy. Soc. Med.* 58(5):295–300.

Hinds, W.H. (1982) "Aerosol Technology: Properties, Behaviors, and Measurement of Airborne Particles" John Wiley and Sons: New York.

Hodgkin, J.E., Abbey, D.E., and Euler, G.L. (1984) "Chronic Obstructive Pulmonary Disease Prevalence in High and Low Photochemical Air Pollution Areas" *Chest* 86:830–838.

Hodkinson, J.R. (1966) "The optical measurement of aerosols" In *Aerosol Science*, Chap. X, edited by C.N. Davies, Academic Press, New York.

Hoek, G., and Brunekreef, B. (1993) "Acute effects of a winter air pollution episode on pulmonary function and respiratory symptoms of children" *Arch. Environ. Health* 48:328–335.

Hoek, G., and Brunekreef, B. (1994) "Effects of low level winter air pollution concentrations on respiratory health of Dutch children" *Environ. Research.* 48:328–335.

Holland, W.W., and Reid, D.D. (1965) "The urban factor in chronic bronchitis" *Lancet* 1:445–448.

Holland, W.W., Bennett, A.E., Cameron, I.R. et al. (1979) "Health effects of particulate pollution: Reappraising the evidence" *Amer. J. Epidemiol.* 110:525–659.

Holma, B. (1989) "Effects of Inhaled Acids on Airway Mucus and Its Consequences For Health. *Environ. Health Perspec.* 79:109.

Horvath S.M. (1985) "Design and measurement considerations for exercise protocols in human air pollution inhalation studies" In *Inhalation Toxicology of Air Pollution: Clinical Research Considerations.* American Society for Testing and Materials, Philadelphia, PA.

Hutzincker, J.J., Johnson, R.L., Shah, J.J., and Cary, R.A. (1982) "Analysis of organic and elemental carbon in ambient aerosols by a thermal-optical method" In *Particulate Carbon: Atmospheric Life Cycles.*, edited by G.T. Wolff and R.L. Klimisch, Plenum Press, New York.

International Commission on Radiological Protection (ICRP) (1966) "Task Force on Lung Dynamics" *Health Physics* 12:173–207.

Ito, K., Kinney, P., and Thurston, G.D. (1995) "Variations in PM_{10} Concentrations within Two Metropolitan Areas and their Implication for Health Effects Analyses" *J. Inhal. Toxicol.* 7(5):735–745.

Ito, K and Thurston, G.D. (1989) "Characterization and Reconstruction of Historical London, England Acidic Aerosol Concentrations" *Environ. Health Perspect.* 79:35.

Ito, K., Thurston, G.D., Hayes, C., and Lippmann, M. (1993) "Associations of London, England, daily mortality with particulate matter, sulfur dioxide, and acidic aerosol pollution" *Arch. Environ. Health* 48:213–220.

Ito, K and Thurston, G.D. (1996) "Daily PM_{10}/mortality associations: an investigation of at-risk populations" *J. Exposure Analysis and Environ. Epidem.* 6:79–96.

Jaenicke, R. (1980) "Atmospheric aerosols and global climate" *J. Aerosol Sci.* 11:577–588.

Janssen, N.A., Hoek, G., Harssema, H., Brunekreef, B. (1995) "A Relationship Between Personal and Ambient PM_{10}" *Epidemiology* 6 (suppl.):S45.

Johnson, K.G., Gideon, R.A. and Loftsgaarden, D.O. (1990) "Montana air pollution study: children's health effects" *Journal Off. Stat.* 5:391–408.

Johansson, T.B., Van Grieken, R.E., Nelson, J.W., and Winchester, J.W. (1975) "Elemental trace analysis of small samples by proton-induced X-ray emission" *Anal. Chem.* 47:855.

Ju, C. and Spengler, J.D., (1981) "Room-to-Room Variations of Concentrations of Respirable Particles in Residences," *Envron. Sci. Technol.* 15:592.

Junge, C.E. (1979) "The importance of mineral dusts as an atmospheric constituent" *Scope Rep.* 14:49–60.

Kemminki K. and Pershagen. G. (1994) "Cancer Risk of Air Pollution: Epidemiological Evidence" *Envir. Health. Perspect.* 102 (Supp 4):187–192.

Kim C.S., Lewars G.A., and Sackner, M.A. (1988) "Measurement of total lung aerosol deposition as an index of lung abnormality" *J. Appl. Physiol.* 64:1527–36.

Kimmel, T.A., Chen, L.C., Bosland, M.C. and Nadziejko, C. (1994) "Effect of Acid Droplet Size on Morphologic Changes in the Rat Lung Following Acute Exposure to O_3 and/or H_2SO_4 Aerosol" *Toxicologist* 14:316.

Kinney P.L., and Özkaynak H. (1991) "Associations of Daily Mortality and Air Pollution in Los Angeles County" *Environ. Research* 54:99–120.

Kinney P.L., Ito, K., and Thurston, G.D. (1995) "A Sensitivity Analysis of Mortality/ PM_{10} Associations in Los Angeles" *Inhalation Toxicol.* 7:59–69.

Knollenberg, R.G., and Luehr, R. (1976) "Open cavity laser active scattering particle spectrometry from 0.05 to 5 m" In *Fine Particles*, edited by B.Y.H. Liu, Academic Press, New York.

Koenig, J.Q., Covert, D.S., and Pierson, W.E. (1989) "Effects of Inhalation of Acidic Compounds of Pulmonary Function in Allergic Adolescent Subjects" *Environ. Health Perspect.* 79:173.

Koenig, J.Q., Larson, T.V., Hanley, Q.S., Rebolledo, V., Dumler, K., et al. (1993) "Pulmonary Function Changes in Children Associated with Fine Particulate Matter" *Environ. Research.* 63:26–38.

Koshal, R.K. and Koshal, M. (1973) "Environments and urban mortality—an econometric approach" *Environ.Poll.* 4:247–269.

Koshal, R.K., and Koshal, M. (1974) "Air Pollution and the respiratory disease mortality in the United States—a quantitative study" *Soc. Indicators Res.* 1:263–278.

Koutrakis, P. "Physico-chemie de l'aerosol urbain: identification et quantification des principales sources par analyse multivariable" *Ph.D. dissertation,* University of Paris.

Koutrakis, P., J. D. Spengler, B. Chang and H. Özkaynak, (1987) "Characterizing Sources of Indoor and Outdoor Aerosols Using PIXE" *Nuclear Instruments and Methods in Physics Research,* B22, p.331.

Koutrakis, P., Wolfson, J.M., Slater, J.L., Brauer, M., and Spengler, J.D. (1988A) "Evaluation of an annular denuder/filter pack system to collect acidic aerosols and gases" *Environ. Sci. and Technol.* 22(12):1463–1468.

Koutrakis, P., Wolfson, J.M., and Spengler, J.D. (1988B) "An improved method for measuring aerosol strong acidity: Results from a ninth-month study in St. Louis, Missouri and Kingston, Tennessee" *Atmos. Environ.* 22(1):157–162.

Koutrakis, P., Wolfson, J.M., Brauer, M., and Spengler, J.D. (1990) "Design of a glass impactor for an annular denuder/filter pack system" *Aerosol Sci. and Technol.* 12:607–613.

Koutrakis P., Thompson K.M., Wolfson J.M., Spengler J.D., Keeler J., and Slater J. (1992) "Determination of aerosol strong acidity losses due to interactions of collected particles: results from laboratory and field studies" *Atmos. Environ.* 26A:987–995.

Koutrakis, P. and Kelly, B.P. (1993) "Equilibrium size of atmospheric aerosol sulfates as a function of particle acidity and ambient relative humidity" *J. Geophys. Res.* 98:7141–7147.

Koutrakis, P., Sioutas, C., Ferguson, S., Wolfson, J.M., Mulik, J.D. and Burton, R.M. (1993) "Development and evaluation of a glass honeycomb denuder/filter pack system to collect atmospheric particles and gases" *Environ. Sci. Technol.* 27:2497–2501.

Lamm, S.H., Hall, T.A., Engel, A., Rueter, F.H., and White, L.D. (1994) "PM_{10} Particulates: AreThey the Major Determinant of Pediatric Respiratory Admissions in Utah County, Utah (1985–1989)?" *Annals of Occupational Hygiene,* 38(1):969–972.

Lannefors, H. and Carlsson, L.E. (1983) "Comparison of some ambient aerosol samplers in combination with PIXE analysis" *X-Ray Spectrometry* 12:138–147.

Last, J.A., Dasgupta, P.K., and Etchison, J.R. (1980) "Inhalation Toxicology of Sodium Sulfite Aerosols in Rats" *Toxicol. Appl. Pharmacol.* 55:229.

Last, J.A., Hyde, D.M., and Chang, D.P.Y.(1984) "A Mechanism of Synergistic Lung Damage by Ozone and a Respirable Aerosol" *Exp. Lung Res.* 7:223.

Last, J.A. (1989) "Effects of Inhaled Acids on Lung Biochemistry" *Environ. Health Perspec.* 79:115.

Lave L.B., and Seskin, E.P. (1970) "Air pollution and human health" *Science* 169:723–733.

Lave, L.B. and E. Seskin (1971) "Health and Air Pollution" *Swedish J. Econ.* 73:76–95.

Lave, L.B. and E. Seskin (1972) "Air Pollution, Climate, and Home Heating: their effects on U.S. Mortality Rates" *Amer. J. Pub. Health* 62:909.

Lave, L.B. and Seskin E.P. (1973) "An Analysis for the Assocation between US Mortality and Air Pollution" *J. Amer. Stat. Assoc.* 68:284–290.

Lave, L.B., and Seskin, E.P. (1977) "Air Pollution and Human Health" *Johns Hopkins University Press*, Baltimore, MD.

Lave, L.B., and Seskin, E.P. (1979) "Epidemiology, causality, and public policy" *American Scientist* 67:178–186.

Lave, L.B. (1982) "Quantitative Risk Assessment in Regulation," *Brookings Institution*, Washington, D.C.

Leaderer, B., Koutrakis, P., Briggs, S., Rizzuto, J. (1990) "Impact of Indoor sources on Residential Aerosol Concentrations" Presented at *Indoor Air '90* in Toronto, ON, Canada. July-August.

Leaderer, B.P., Koutrakis, P., Briggs, S.L.K. and Rizzuto, J. (1994) "The Mass Concentration and Elemental Composition of Indoor Aerosols in Suffolk and Onondaga Counties, New York," *Indoor Air* 4:23.

Lebowitz, M.D., Holberg, C.J., Boyer, B., and Hayes, C. (1985) "Respiratory symptoms and peak flow associated with indoor and outdoor air pollutants in the southwest" *J. Air Poll. Control Assoc.* 35:1154–1158.

Lebret, E. (1990) "Errors in Exposure Measures" *Toxicology and Industrial Health* 6:147–156.

Leikauf, G., Yeates, D.B., Wales, K.A., et al. (1981) "Effects of Inhaled Sulfuric Acid Aerosol on Respiratory Mechanics and Mucociliary Particle Clearance in Healthy Nonsmoking Adults" *Amer. Ind. Hyg. Assoc. J.* 42:273.

Leonard, A.G., Crowley, D., and Benton, J. (1950) "Atmospheric Pollution in Dublin during the years 1944–1950" *Roy. Dub. Soc. Sci. Proc.* 25:166–167.

Liang K.Y. and Zeger S.L. (1984) "Longitudinal data analysis using generalized linear models" *Biometrika* 73:13–22.

Lin, C.I., Baker, M., and Charlson, R.J. (1973) "Absorption coefficient of atmospheric aerosols: a method for measurement" *Appl. Opt.* 12:1356.

Linton, R.W., Loh. A., Natusch, D.F.S., Evans, C.A., and Williams, P.(1976) "Surface Predominance of Trace Elements in Airborne Particles" *Science* 191:8852.

Lioy, P.J. (1990) "Assessing Total Human Exposure to Contaminants" *Environ. Sci. Tech.* 24:938–945.

Lioy, P.J. and Waldman, J.M. (1989) "Acidic Sulfate Aerosols: Characterization and Exposure" *Environ. Health Perspect.* 79:15.

Lioy, P.J., M. Avdenko, Harkov R., Atherholt, T., and Daisey, J.M. (1985) "A Pilot Indoor-Outdoor Study of Organic Particulate Matter and Particulate Mutagenicity," *J. Air Poll. Control Assoc.* 35:653.

Lioy, P.J., Waldman, J.M. Buckley, T., Butler, J., and Piearinen, C. (1990) "The Personal, Indoor and Outdoor Concentrations of PM_{10} Measured in an Industrial Community during the Winter," *Atmos. Environ.* 24B(1):576.

Lipfert, F, Malone, R.G., Daum, M.L. et al.(1988)"A Statistical Study of Macroepidemiology of Air Pollution and Total Mortality" Report for US DOE.

Lipfert, F.W. (1984) "Air pollution and mortality: Specification searches using SMSA-based data" *J. Environ. Econ. Manage.* 11:208–243.

Lipfert, F.W. (1994) "Air Pollution and Community Health: A Critical Review and Data Sourcebook" *Van Nostrand Reinhold:* New York, pp.556.

Lipfert, F.W. and Hammerstrom, T. (1992) "Temporal patterns in air pollution and hospital admissions" *Environ. Research.* 59:374–399.

Lipfert, F.W., Malone, R.G., Daum, M.L., Mendell, N.R., and Yang, C.C. (1988) "A Statistical Study of the Macroepidemiology of Air Pollution and Total Mortality" Prepared for the *Office of Environmental Analysis.* U.S. Department of Energy.

Lipfert, F.W. and Wyzga, R.E. (1995a) "Uncertainties in Identifying Responsible Pollutants in Observational Epidemiological Studies" *Inhal. Toxicol.* 7:671–689.

Lipfert, F.W. and Wyzga, R.E. (1995b) "Air Pollution and Mortality: Issues and Uncertainties" *J. Air Waste Manage. Assoc.* 45:949–966.

Lippmann, M. and Altshuler, B. (1976) "Regional Deposition of Aerosols" In *Air Pollution and the Lung,* pp 25–48. E.F. Aharanson, A. Ben-David and H.A. Klingberg, Eds. Halsted-Wiley. Jerusalem.

Lippmann, M. and Ito, K., (1995) "Separating the Effects of Temperature and Season on Dialy Mortality from those of Air Pollution in London: 1965–1972" *Inhal. Toxicol.* 7:85–87.

Lippmann, M. and Lioy, P.J (1985) "Critical Issues in Air Pollution Epidemiology" *Envir. Health Perspec.* 62:243–258.

Lippmann, M, Schlesinger, R.B., Leikauf, G., et al. (1982) "Effects of Sulphuric Acid Aerosols on Respiratory Tract Airways" *Ann. Occup. Hyg.* 26:677.

Lippmann, M, Gearhart, J.M., and Schlesinger, R.B.(1987) "Basis For a Particle Size-Selective TLV for Sulfuric Acid Aerosols" *Appl. Ind. Hyg.* 2:188.

Lippmann, M. (1989) "Sampling aerosols by filtration" In *Air Sampling Instruments,* edited by S.V. Hering. American Conference of Governmental Industrial Hygienists, Inc., Cincinnati, OH.

Liu, B.Y.H. and Pui, D.Y.H. (1975) "Unipolar charging of aerosol particles in the continuum regime" *J.Aerosol Sci.* 6:249.

Liu, B.C. and Yu, E.S.H. (1976) "Physical and economic damage functions for air pollutants by receptor" EPA-600/5–76-011, *U.S. Environmental Protection Agency,* Corvallis, Oregon.

Liu, B.C., and Yu, E.S.H. (1977) "Mortality and air pollution revisited" *J. Air Poll. Control Assoc.* 26:968–971.

Lodge, J. P. (1969) "The Smoake of London: Two Prophecies" Maxwell Reprint Company, Elmsford, London.

Logan, W.P.D., (1953) "Mortality in London fog incident" *Lancet* 1:336–338.

Loo, B.W., Jacklevic, J.M., and Goulding, F.S. (1976) "Dichotomous sampler for large-scale monitoring of airborne particulate matter" In *Fine Particles,* edited by B.Y.H. Liu, Academic Press, New York.

Lungdren, D. et al. (1976) "Aerosol mass measurements using piezoelectric crystal sensors" In *Fine Particles,* edited by B.Y.H. Liu, Academic Press, New York.

Lutz, L.J., (1983) "Health effects of air pollution measured by outpatient visits" *J. Fam. Pract.* 16:307–313.

McIlvaine C.M. (1994) "Development of the MAP-O₃ Ozone Model for Predicting Seasonal Average Ozone Cocentrations Due to Large Point Source NO_x Emissions" *Ph. D. Dissertation.* University of Tennessee, Knoxville, TN.

Macias, E.S. and Husar, R.B. (1976) "A review of atmospheric particulate measurement via beta attenuation technique" In *Fine Particles*, edited by B.Y.H. Liu, Academic Press, New York.

Mage, D.T. (1995) "The Relationship Between Total Suspended Particulate Matter (TSP) and British Smoke Measurements in London: Development of a Simple Model" *J. Air Waste Manage. Assoc.* 45:737–739.

Mage, D.T. and Buckley, T.J., (1995) "The Relationship between Personal Exposures and Ambient Concentrations of Particulate Matter" Paper No. 95-MP18.01 Presented at the 88th Annual Meeting of the Air and Waste Management Association. June 18–23, San Antonio, TX.

Marple, V.A. and Liu, B.Y.H. (1974) "Characteristics of laminar jet impactors" *Environ. Sci. Technol.* 7:648–654.

Marple, V.A. and Willeke, K. (1976) In *Fine Particles: Aerosol generation, measurement, sampling, and analysis,* edited by B.Y.H Liu, Academic Press, New York.

Marple, V.A., and Chien, C. (1980) "Virtual impactors: a theoretical study" *Environ. Sci. Technol.* 8:976–985.

Marple V.A., Rubow K.L. and Behm, S.M. (1991) "A micro-orifice uniform deposit impactor (MOUDI)" *Aerosol Sci. & Technol.* 14:434–446.

Martin, A.E. (1964) "Mortality and morbidity statistics and air pollution" *Proc. Roy. Soc. Med.* 57:969–975.

Masuda, H., Hochrainer, D., and Stober, W. (1988) "An improved virtual impactor for particle classification and generation of test aerosols with narrow size distributions" *J. Aerosol Sci.* 10:275–287.

McCarroll J. (1979) "Health Effects Associated with Increased Use of Coal" *Air Pollution Control Association* 72nd Ann. mtg, Cincinnati, OH.

McCarthy, J.F., Yurek, G.J., Elliot, J.F., and Amdur, M.O. (1982) "Generation and Characterization of Submicron Aerosols of Zinc Oxide" *Amer. Ind. Hyg. Assoc. J.* 43:880.

McDow, S.R., and Hutzincker, J.J. (1990) "Vapor adsorption artifact in the sampling of organic aerosols: face velocity effects" *Atmos. Environ.* 24A:2563–2571.

McMurry P.H. and Zhang X.Q. (1989) "Size distribution of ambient organic and elemental carbon" *Aerosol Sci. & Technol.* 10:430–437.

Mattson, M.E., Pollack, E.S. and Cullen, J.W. (1987) "What are the Odds that Smoking will Kill You?" *Amer. J. Public Health,* 77, 425–431.

Miller, P.D., Ainsworth, D., Lam, H.F. and Amdur, M.O. (1987) "Effect of Ozone Exposure on Lung Functions and Plasma Protoglandin and Thromboxane Concentrations in Guinea Pigs" *Toxicol. Appl. Pharmacol.* 88:132.

Miller F.J, Angilvel S., Menache M.G., et al. (1995) "Dosimetric issues related to particulate toxicity" *Inhal. Toxicol.* 7:615–32.

Moolgavkar S.H., Luebeck E.G., Hall T.A, et al. (1985) "Particulate air pollution, sulfur dioxide, and daily mortality: A reanalysis of the Steubenville Data" *Inhal. Toxicol.* 7:35–44.

Moolgavkar S.H. and Luebeck E.G. (1996) "A Critical Review of the Evidence on Particles Air Pollution and Mortality" *Epidemiology* 7:420–428.

Morgan, M.G.; S.C. Morris; A.K. Meir; and D.L. Shenk. (1978a) "A probabilistic methodology for estimating air pollution effects from coal-fired power plants" *Energy Systems and Policy* 2:287–310.

Morgan, M.G., Morris, S.C., Meir, A.K., and Shenk, D.L. (1978b) "Sulfur control in coal-fired power plants: a probabilistic approach to policy analysis" *J. Air Poll. Control Assoc.* 28:993–97.

Morgan M.G, Morris, S.C., Henrion A., Amurai D.A.L., and Rush W.R. (1984) "Technical Uncertainty in Quantitative Policy Analyses: a Sulfur Pollution Example" *Risk Analysis* 4:201.

Morrow P.E., Utell M.J., Bauer M.A., et al. (1994) "Effects of near ambient levels of sulfuric acid aerosol on lung function in exercising subjects with asthma and COPD" *Ann. Occup. Hyg.* 38(Suppl):933–8.

Morrow P.E., and Utell M.J. (1995) "Effects of near ambient levels of sulfuric acid aerosol on lung function in exercising subjects with asthma and COPD" *Ann. Occup. Hyg.*

Murray, D.M. and Burmaster, D.E. (1995) "Residential Air Exchange Rates in the United States: Empirical and Estimated Parametric Distributions by Season and Climatic Region" *Risk Analysis* 15:459–465.

Mulik, J., Puckett, R, Williams, D., and Sawicki, E. (1976) "Ion chromatographic analysis of sulfate and nitrate in ambient aerosols" *Anal. Lett.* 9:653.

National Center for Health Statistics (1985) "Vital Statistics of the United States, 1980, Volume II, Annual Mortality Part B" *U.S. Government Printing Office, Washington, D.C.*

Neas, L.M., Dockery, D.W., Spengler, J.D., Speizer, F.E., and Tollerud, D.J. (1992) "The association of ambient air pollution with twice daily peak expiratory flow measurements in children" *Amer. Rev. Resp. Disease* 145(4):A429.

Novakov, T., Mueller, P.K., Alcoer, A.E. and Vtvos, J.W. (1972) "Chemical Composition of Pasadena Aerosol by Particle Size and Time of Day: III. Chemical States of Nitrogen and Sulfur by Photoelectron Spectroscopy" *J. Colloid Interface Sci.* 30:225.

Öberd rster G., Soderholm S.C. and Finkelstein, J., (1992) "Role of Alveolar Macrophages in Lung Injury: Studies with Ultrafine PArticles" *Envir. Health Perspect.* 97:193.

Öberd rster, G., Gelein, R.M., Ferin, J., and Weiss, B. (1995) "Association of particulate air pollution and acute mortality: Involvement of ultrafine particles?" *Inhal. Toxicol.* 7:111–24.

Öberdorster G. (1996) "Effects of ultrafine particles in the lung and potential relevance to environmental particles" In *Proceedings of the 1995 Warsaw Particle Workshop*, Delft University Press, Delft, Poland.

O'Connor, G. (1996) Personal communication with George O'Connor, Boston University School of Medicine.

OECD (Organization for Economic Cooperation and Development) (1974) "Seminar on Problems in Transfrontier Pollution" Paris, January.

OECD (1977) "The Organization for Economic Cooperation and Development programme on long range transport of air pollution: measurements and findings" Paris.

Office of Smoking and Health (1979) "Smoking and Health. A Report of the Surgeon General" U.S. Department of Health, Education, and Welfare, Public Health Service, Office of Smoking and Health. DHEW Publication No.(PHS) 79–50066.

Osebold, J.W., Gershwin, L.J. and Zee, Y.C. (1980) "Studies on the Enhancement of Allergic Lung Sensitization by Inhalation of Ozone and Sulfuric Acid Aerosol" *J. Environ. Path. Toxocol.* 3:221.

Osornio-Vargas, A.H., Alfara-Moreno, E., Rosas, J., Lindroos, P.M., Badgett, A., Dreher, K., and Bonner, J.C. (1996) "The *in vitro* Toxicity of Ambient PM_{10} Particles from the Southern, Central Regions of Mexico City to Lung Fibroblasts is Related to Transition Metal Content" *Amer. J. Respir. Crit. Care Med.* 153:A15.

Ostro, B.D. (1983) "The effects of air pollution on work loss and morbidity" *J. Environ. Econ. Manage.* 10:371–382.

Ostro, B.D. (1984) "A search for a threshold in the relationship of air pollution to mortality: A reanalysis of data on London winters" *Environ. Health Perspect.* 58:397–399.

Ostro, B.D. (1987) "Air pollution and morbidity revisited: A specification test" *J. Environ. Econ. Manage.* 14:87–98.

Ostro, B.D. (1990) "Associations between morbidity and alternative measures of particulate matter" *Risk Analysis* 10:421–427.

Ostro, B.D. (1993) "The association of air pollution and mortality: examining the case for inference" *Arch. Environ. Health* Vol 48, pp.336–342.

Ostro, B.D., and Rothschild, S. (1989) "Air pollution and acute respiratory morbidity: An observational study of multiple pollutants" *Environ. Research* 50:238–247.

Ostro, B.D., Lipsett, M.J., Wiener, M.B., and Selner, J.C. (1991) "Asthmatic response to airborne acid aerosols" *Amer. J. Public Health* 81:694–702.

Ostro, B.D., Lipsett, M.J., Mann, J.K., Krupnick, A., and Harrington, W. (1993) "Air pollution and respiratory morbidity among adults in Southern California" *Amer. J. Epidemiol.* 137:691–700.

Ostro, B.D., et al. (1995) To be published.

Ostro, B.D., Sanchez, J.N., Aranda, C., and Eskeland, G.S. (1996) "Air Pollution and Mortality: Results from a Study of Santiago, Chile" *J. Expos. Anal. Environ. Epidemiol.* 6:97–114.

Ott, W. (1985) "Total human exposure" *Environ. Sci. Tech.* 19:880–885.

Ott, W., Thomas, J., Mage, D., and Wallace, L. (1988) "Validation of the simulation of human activity and pollutant exposure (SHAPE) model using paired days from the Denver, CO, carbon monoxide field study" *Atmos. Environ.* 22:2101–2113.

Özkaynak, H., and Thurston, G.D. (1987) "Associations between 1980 U.S. mortality rates and alternative measures of airborne particle concentration" *Risk Analysis.* 7:449–461.

Özkaynak, H., Spengler J.D., Butler, D.A., and Billick, I.H. (1993) "Predicting the distribution of population exposures to NO_2 in a large urban area" Presented at *Indoor Air '93*, Helsinki, Finland, July.

Özkaynak, H., Xue, J., Zhou, H., Spengler, J., and Thurston, G.D. (1996a) "Inter-community Differences in Acid Aerosol (H^+/SO_4^{2-})" *J. Expos. Anal. Environ. Epidemiol.* 6(1):35–55.

Özkaynak, H., Xue, J., Spengler, J., Wallace, L., Pellizzari, E., and Jenkins, P. (1996b) "Personal Exposure to Airborne Particles and Metals: Results from the Particle Team Study in Riverside, California" *J. Expos. Anal. Environ. Epidemiol.* 6:57–78.

Özkaynak, H., Spengler, J.D., Ludwig, J.F, Butler, D.A., Clayton, C.A. and Wiener, R.W. (1990) "Personal Exposure to Particulate Matter: Findings from the Particle Total Exposure Assessment Methodology (PTEAM) Prepilot Study" *Proc. Fifth International Conference on Indoor Air Quality and Climate* 2:571, Toronto.

Özkaynak, H. (1993) "Review of Recent Epidemiological Data on Health Effects of Particles, Ozone, and Nitrogen Dioxide" Presented at the National Association for Clean Air Conference, "Clean Air Challenges in a Changing South Africa," Brits, South Africa, November.

Özkaynak, H., Xue, J., Spengler, J., Pellizzari, E. and Jenkins, P. (1994) "Personal Exposure to Airborne Particles and Metals: Results from the Particle TEAM Study in Riverside, California" Presented at the *ISEE/ISEA Joint Conference at Research Triangle Park*, NC, September 12–21.

Özkaynak, H., Xue, J., Weker, R., Butler, D., Koutrakis, P. and Spengler, J. (1995) "The Particle TEAM (PTEAM) Study: Analysis of Data," Vol. III, Final Report to the Environmental Protection Agency, Research Triangle Park, NC..

Palmgren, U, Strom, G., Blomquist G., and Malmberg, P. (1986) "Collection of airborne microorganisms on nuclepore filter; estimation and analysis-EAMNEA Method" *J. Appl. Bacteriol.* 61:401.

Pasquill, F. (1961) "The estimation of the dispersion of windborn materials" *Meteorology Mag.* 90:1963.

Pasquill, F. (1962) "Atmospheric Diffusion" *Van Nostrand Reinhold*, Princeton, New Jersey.

Pataschnick, H. and Rupprecht, E.G. "Continuous PM_{10} measurements using the tapered element oscillating microbalance" *J. Air Waste Manage. Assoc.* 41:1079–1083.

Pechan, P.M. and Associates (1994) "National PM study: OPPE Particulate Programs Evaluation System" report to US Environmental Protection Agency (with 1996 update).

Pierson, W.R., Brachaczek, W.W., Truex, T.J., Butler, J.W., and Korniski, T.J.M, (1980) "Ambient sulfate measurements on Allegheny Mountain and the question of atmospheric sulfate in the northeastern United States" *Ann. N.Y. Acad. Sci.*, 338, 145–173.

Pitts and Metcalf, eds. (1969) "Advances in Environmental Science" *Wiley-Interscience* 1:8, NY.

Plantagenet, E. (1307) "Letter to the Sheriff of Surrey" Quoted and translated by Sir W. Hawthorne, in "Energy and environment, conflict or compromise" Trueman Wood Lecture, *J. Roy. Soc. Arts,* July 1978.

Pope, C.A. III. (1989) "Respiratory disease associated with community air pollution and a steel mill, Utah Valley" *Amer. J. Public Health* 79:623–628.

Pope, C.A. III. (1991) "Respiratory hospital admissions associated with PM$_{10}$ pollution in Utah, Salt Lake, and Cache Valleys" *Arch. Environ. Health* 46:90–97.

Pope, C.A. III, Dockery, D.W., Spengler, J.D., and Raizenne, M.E. (1991) "Respiratory health and PM$_{10}$ pollution: A daily time series analysis" *Amer. Rev. Resp. Disease* 144:668–674.

Pope, C.A. III and Dockery, D.W. (1992) "Acute health effects of PM$_{10}$ pollution on symptomatic and asymptomatic children" *Amer. Rev. Resp. Disease* 145:1123–1128.

Pope, C.A. III, Schwartz J, and Ransom MR. (1992) "Daily mortality and PM$_{10}$ pollution in Utah Valley" *Arch. Environ. Health* 47:211–17.

Pope, C.A. III, and Kanner, R.E. (1993) "Acute effects of PM$_{10}$ pollution on pulmonary function of smokers with mild to moderate chronic obstructive pulmonary disease" *Amer. Rev. Resp. Disease.* 147:1336–1340.

Pope, C.A. III (1996a) "Epidemiology Investigations of the Health Effects of Particulate Air Pollution: Strengths and Limitations" Presented at 2nd Colloquium on Particulate Air Pollution and Health, Park City, Utah, *Appl. Occup. Environ. Hygiene* (submitted).

Pope, C.A.III (1996b) "Combustion-Source Particulate Air Pollution and Human Health: Causal Associations or Confounding?" in *"Particulate Matter: Health and Regulatory Issues"* VIP-49 Pittsburgh, PA. April 4–6, 1995.

Pope, C.A. III and Kanner, R.E. (1993) "Acute effects of PM$_{10}$ pollution on pulmonary function of smokers with mild to moderate chronic obstructive pulmonary disease" *Amer. Rev. Resp. Disease* 147:1336–1340.

Pope, C.A. III, Schwartz, J., and Ransom, M.R. (1992) "Daily mortality and PM$_{10}$ pollution in Utah Valley" *Arch. Environ. Health.* 47:211–217.

Pope C.A. III, Dockery D.W. and Schwartz J. (1995a) "Review of epidemiological evidence of health effects of particulate air pollution" *Inhal. Toxicol.* 7:1–18.

Pope, C.A. III, Bates, D.V., and Raizenne, M.E. (1995b) "Health effects of particulate air pollution: Time for reassessment?" *Environ. Health Perspect.* 103:472–480.

Pope, C.A. III, Thun, M.J., Namboodiri, M.M., Dockery, D.W., Evans, J.S., Speizer, F.E. and Heath, C.W. (1995) "Particulate air pollution as a predictor of mortality in a prospective study of U.S. adults" *Amer. J. Resp. Crit. Care Med.* 151:669–674.

Pope, C.A. III, and Schwartz, J. (1996) "Time Series for the Analysis of Pulmonary Health Data" *Amer. J. Resp. Crit. Care Med.* (in press).

Pope, C.A III, and Kalkstein, L.S. (1996) "Synoptic weather modelling and estimates of the exposure response relationship between daily mortality and particulate air pollution" *Environ. Health Perspect.* 104:414–420.

Portney, P.R., and Mullahy, J. (1990) "Urban air quality and chronic respiratory disease" *Regional Sci. Urban Econ.* 20:407–418.

Possanzini M., Febo A., and Liberti, A. (1983) "New Design of High Performance Denuder for the Sampling of Atmospheric Pollutants" *Atmos. Environ.* 17:2605–2610.

Prichard, R.J., Ghio, A.J., Lehmann, J.R., Winsett, D.W., Tepper, J.F., Park, P., Gilmour, M.I., Dreher, K.L., and Costa, D.A. (1996) "Oxidant Generation and Lung Injury after Particulate Air Pollutant Exposure Increase with the Concentrations of Associated Metals" *Inhal. Toxicol.* (In Press).

Prichard, R.J. and Ghio, A.J. (1995) "Humic Acid-Like Substances are Present in Air Pollution Particles" *Amer. J. Respir. Crit. Care Med.* 151:A840.

Prospero, J.M, Charlson, R.J., Mohnen, V., Jaenicke, R., Delany, A.C., Moyers, J., Zoller, W., and Rahn, K. (1983) "The atmospheric aerosol system: an overview" *Rev. Geophysics and Space Physics* 21:1607–1629.

Quackenboss, J.J., Krzyzanowski, M., and Lebowitz, M.D. (1991) "Exposure Assessment Approaches to Evaluate Respiratory Health Effects of Particulate Matter and Nitrogen Dioxide" *J. Exposure Anal. Environ. Epidemiol.* 1:83–107.

Quann, R.J., Neville, M., Janghorbani, M., Mims, C.A., and Sarofim, A.F. (1982) "Mineral Matter and Trace Element Vaporization in a Laboratory Pulverized Coal Combustion System" *Environ. Sci. Technol.* 16:776.

Rahn, K.A. (1981) "The Mn/V ratio as a tracer of large-scale sources of pollution aerosol for the Arctic" *Atmos. Environ.* 15:1457–1464.

Raizenne M.E., Burnett R.T., Stern B., et al. (1989) "Acute lung function responses to ambient acid aerosol exposures in children" *Environ. Health Perspect.* 79:179–85.

Raizenne, M., Neas, L., Damokosh, A., Dockberg, D., Spengler, J., Koutrakis, P., Ware, J., and Speizer, F. (1993) "Health effects of acid aerosols on North American children: Pulmonary function" Paper presented at the *American Lung Association/American Thoracic Society International Conference*, San Francisco, CA, May 16–19.

Raizenne, M., Neas, L.M., Damokosh, A.I., Dockery, D.W., Spengler, J.D., Koutrakis, P., Ware, J.H. and Speizer, F.E. (1996) "Health Effects of Acid Aerosols on North American Children: Pulmonary Function" *Environ. Health Perspect.* 104:506–514.

Ransom, M.R., and Pope, C.A. III. (1992) "Elementary school absences and PM_{10} pollution in Utah Valley" *Environ. Research* 58:204–219.

Repace, J.L., and Lowery, A.H. (1980) "Indoor Air Pollution, Tobacco Smoke, and Public Health" *Science* 208:464–472.

Risby, T.H. Ed. (1979) "Ultratrace Metal Analysis in Biological Sciences and Environment" *Advances in Chemistry* Series 172, Amer. Chem. Soc., Washington, DC.

Robinson, J. and Nelson, W.C. (1995) "National Human Activity Pattern Survey Data Base" Research Triangle Park, NC: *U.S. Environmental Protection Agency.*

Roemer, W., Hoek, G., and Brunekreef, B. (1993) "Effect of ambient winter air pollution on respiratory health of children with chronic respiratory symptoms" *Amer. Rev. Resp. Disease.* 147:118–124.

Romero, F., and Elejalde, C. (1982) "Heavy metal contamination of soils at Biscay" in *Analytical Techniques in Environmental Chemistry.*, edited by J. Albaiges, Pergamon Press, Oxford.

Ross, F.F., and T.T. Frankenberg (1971) "What sulphur dioxide problem?" *Combustion*, August, p. 6.

Ryan, P. Barry (1991) "An Overview of Human Exposure Modeling" *J. Expos. Anal. Environ. Epidemiol.* 1:453–473.

Saldiva, P.H.N., Pope, C.A. III, Schwartz, J., Dockery, D.W., Lichtenfels, A.J., Salge, J.M., Barone, I., and Bohm, G.M. (1995) "Air pollution and mortality in elderly people: A time series study in Sao Paulo, Brazil" *Arch. Environ. Health.* 50:159–163.

Saltzman, B.E. (1984) "Generalized performance characteristics of miniature cyclones for respirable aerosol sampling" *Amer. Ind. Hyg. Assoc. J.* 45:671.

Samet J.M. (1996) "Issues in the selection of subjects for clinical and epidemiological studies of asthma" In *Susceptibility to inhaled pollutants*, M.J.Utell and R.Frank, Eds. 1989, American Society for Testing and Materials; Philadephia, PA.

Samet, J.M., Zeger, S.L. and Berhane, K. (1995) "The association of mortality and particulate air pollution" In *Particulate Air Pollution and Daily Mortality: Replication and Validation of Selected Studies.* Prepared by the Health Effects Institute, Cambridge, MA.

Samet, J.M., Speizer, F.E., Bishop, Y., Spengler, J.D., and Ferris, B.G., Jr. (1981) "The relationship between air pollution and emergency room visits in an industrial community" *J. Air Poll. Control Assoc.* 31:236–240.

Samet, J.M., Zeger, S.L., Kelsall, J.E., Xu, J. and Kalkstein, L.S. (1996) "Weather, air pollution and mortality in Philadelphia, 1973–1980" Report to Health Effects Institute, Cambridge, MA.

Sandstrom, T., and Rudell, B. (1991) "Bronchoalveolar neutrophilia and depressed macrophage phagosytosis following single-exposure to diesel exhaust" *Amer. Rev. Respir. Disease* 143:A96 [Abstract].

Santanam, S., Spengler, J.D., Ryan, P.B. (1990) "Particulate Matter Exposures Estimated from an Indoor-Outdoor Source Apportionment Study" Presented at *Indoor Air '90* in Toronto, ON, Canada. July–August.

Schenker, M B., Speizer, F.E., Samet, J.M., et al. (1983) "Health Effects of Air Pollution Due to Coal Combustion in the Chestnut Ridge Region of Pennsylvania: Results of Cross-Sectional Analysis in Adults" *Arch. Environ. Health* 38:325.

Schlesinger, R.B, Halpern, M., Albert, R.E.and Lippmann, M. (1979) "Effect of Chronic Inhalation of Sulfuric Acid Upon Mucociliary Clearance from the Lungs of Donkeys" *J. Environ. Pathol. Toxicol.* 2:1351.

Schlesinger, R.B., Lippmann, M. and Albert, R.E.: "Effects of Short-Term Exposure to Sulfuric Acid and Ammonium Sulfate Aerosols Upon Bronchial Airway Function in the Donkey"*Amer. Ind. Hyg. Assoc. J.* 39:275.

Schlesinger, R.B., Chen, L.C., and Driscoll, K.E. (1984) "Exposure-Response Relationship of Bronchial Mucociliary Clearance in Rabbits Following Acute Inhalations of Sulfuric Acid" *Toxicology Letters* 22:249.

Schlesinger, R.B., Zelikoff, J.T., Chen, L.C. and Kinney, P.L. (1992a) "Assessment of Toxicologic Interactions Resulting from Acute Inhalation Exposure to Sulfuric Acid and Ozone Mixtures" *Toxicol. Appl. Pharm.* 115:183.

Schlesinger, R.B., Gorczynski, J.E., Dennison, J., Richards, L., Kinney, P.L., and Bosland, M.C. (1992b) "Long-Term Intermittent Exposure to Sulfuric Acid Aerosol, Ozone, and Their Combination: Alterations in Tracheobronchial Mucociliary Clearancxe and Epithelial Secretory Cells" *Exp. Lung Res.* 18:505.

Schlesinger, R.B. (1995) "Toxicological Evidence For Health Effects From Inhaled Particulate Pollution: Does It Support the Human Experience?" *Inhal. Toxicol.* 7:99–109.

Schlesinger, R.B., McGovern, T. and El-Fawal, H.A.N. (1993) "Nonspecific Bronchial Responsiveness Assessed *in Vitro* Following Acute Inhalation Exposure to Ozone and Ozone/Sulfuric Acid Mixtures" *Exp. Lung Res.* 21:129.

Schrenk, H.H., Heiman, H., Clayton, G.D. et al. (1949) "Air Pollution in Donora, PA, Epidemiology of the Unusual Smog Episode of October 1948" U.S. *Public Health Bulletin* No. 306. U.S. Government Printing Office, Washington, DC.

Schuetzle, D., Cronn, D., Crittenden, A.L., and Charlson, R.J. (1975) "Molecular composition of secondary aerosol and its possible origin" *Environ. Sci. Technol.* 9:838.

Schwartz, J. (1989) "Lung function and chronic exposure to air pollution: A cross-sectional analysis of NHANES II" *Environ. Research* 50:309–321.

Schwartz, J. (1991) "Particulate air pollution and daily mortality in Detroit" *Environ. Research* 56:204–213.

Schwartz J. (1993a) "Air pollution and daily mortality in Birmingham, Alabama" *Amer. J. Epidemiol.* 137:1136 47.

Schwartz, J. (1993b) "Particulate Air Pollution and Chronic Respiratory Disease" *Environ. Research* 62:7.

Schwartz, J. (1994a) "Air pollution and hospital admissions for the elderly in Birmingham, AL" *Amer. J. Epidemiol.* 139:589–590.

Schwartz, J. (1994b) "Particulate air pollution and chronic respiratory disease" *Environ. Research* 62:7–13.

Schwartz, J. (1994c) "What are people dying of on high air pollution days?" *Environ. Research* 64:26–35.

Schwartz, J. (1994d) "PM_{10}, Ozone, and Hospital Admissions for the elderly in Minneapolis-St. Paul" *Arch. Environ. Health* 49:366–374.

Schwartz, J. (1994e) "Air pollution and daily mortality: a review and meta analysis" *Environ. Research* 64:36–52.

Schwartz, J. (1994f) "Particulate air pollution and daily mortality in Cincinnati, Ohio" *Environ. Health Perspect.* 102:186–189.

Schwartz, J. (1994g) "Air pollution and hospital admissions for the elderly in Detroit" *Amer. J. Resp. Crit. Care Med.* 150:648–655.

Schwartz, J. (1996) "Health Effects of Air Pollution From Traffic: Ozone and Particulate Matter" *Health at the Crossroads* 1–24.

Schwartz, J., and Dockery, D.W. (1992a) "Increased mortality in Philadelphia associated with daily air pollution concentrations" *Amer. Rev. Resp. Disease* 145:600–604.

Schwartz, J., and Dockery D.W. (1992b) "Particulate air pollution and daily mortality in Steubenville, Ohio" *Amer. J. Epidemiol.* 135:12–19.

Schwartz, J., and Marcus, A. (1990) "Mortality and air pollution in London: A time series analysis" *Amer. J. Epidemiol.* 131:185–194.

Schwartz, J., Spix, C., Wichmann, H.E., and Malin, E. (1991) "Air pollution and acute respiratory illness in five German communities" *Environ. Research* 56:1–14.

Schwartz, J., Slater, D., Larson, T.V., Pierson, W.E., and Koenig, J.Q. (1993) "Particulate air pollution and hospital emergency visits for asthma in Seattle" *Amer. Rev. Resp. Disease* 147:826–831.

Schwartz, G.P., Daisey, J.M., and Lioy, P.J. (1981) "Effect of sampling duration on the concentration of particulate organics collected on glass fiber filters" *Amer. Ind. Hyg. Assoc. J.*, 41:258–263.

Schwartz, J., Dockery, D.W., Neas, L.M., Wypij, D., Ware, J.H., Spengler, J.D., Koutrakis, P., Speizer, F.E., and Ferris, B.G. (1994) "Acute effects of summer air pollution on respiratory symptom reporting in children" *Amer. J. Respir. Crit. Care Med.* 150:124–1242.

Schwartz, J., Dockery, D.W. and Neas, L.M. (1996) "Is daily mortality associated specifically with fine particles" *J.Air Waste Manage. Assoc.* (In press).

Seaton A., MacNee W., Donaldson K, and Godden D. (1995) "Particulate air pollution and acute health effects" *Lancet* 345:176–8.

Sexton, K. and Ryan, B. (1988) "Assessment of Human Exposure to Air Pollution: Methods, Measurements and Models," In *Air Pollution, the Automobile and Public Health,* Health Effects Institute, National Academy Press, Washington, DC.

Shaw, R.W., Stevens, R.K., Bowermaster, J., Tesch, J.W. and Tew, E. (1982) "Measurements of atmospheric nitrate and nitric acid: the denuder difference experiment" *Atmos. Environ.* 16:845.

Sheldon, L.S., Hartwell, T.D., Cox, B.G., Sickles II, J.E., Pellizzari, E.D., Smith, M.L., Perritt, R.L., and Jones, S.M. (1989) "An investigation of infiltration and indoor air quality" Final Report. NY State ERDA Contract No. 736-CON-BCS-85. New York State Energy Research and Development Authority, Albany, NY.

Sheppard, D.(1988) "Sulfur Dioxide and Asthma: A Double Edged Sword?" *J. Allergy Clin. Immunol.* 82:961.

Sehnert, Long and Risby (1996) (in press.).

Shprentz, D.S. Bryner, G.C., and Shprentz J.S., (1996) "Breath Taking: Premature Mortality due to Particle Air Pollution in 239 American Cities" *National Resources Defense Council* (NRDC), New York, NY.

Shy, C.M. (1979) "Epidemiologic evidence and the United States air quality standards" *Amer. J. Epidemiol.* 110:661–671.

Sioutas, C., Koutrakis, P., and Burton, R.M. (1994) "Development of a low cutpoint slit virtual impactor for sampling ambient fine particles" *J. Aerosol Sci.* 25:1321–1330.

Sorlie, P.D., Kannel, W.B. and O'Connor, G. (1989) "Mortality associated with respiratory function and symptoms in advanced age" *Amer. Rev. Respir. Disease* 140:379–384.

Speizer, F.E. (1989) "The rise in chronic obstructive pulmonary disease mortality. Overview and summary" *Amer. Rev. Resp. Disease* 140:S106-7.

Spektor D.M. and Yen B.M. (1989) "Effect of concentration and cumulative exposure of inhaled sulfuric acid on tracheobronchial particle clearance in healthy humans" *Environ. Health Perspect.* 79:167–72.

Spengler, J. (1995) "The Particle TEAM (PTEAM) Study: Analysis of Data" *Final Report to the Environmental Protection Agency*, Research Triangle Park, NC. V. 3.

Spengler, J.D., Brauer, M. and Koulvakis, P. (1990) "Acid Air and Health" *Environ. Sci. Tech.* 24(7):946–955.

Spengler, J. D., D. W. Dockery, W. A. Turner, J. M. Wolfson and B. G. Ferris, Jr., (1981) "Long-Term Measurements of Respirable Sulfates and Particles Inside and Outside Homes" *Atmos. Environ.* 15:23.

Spengler, J.D., Keeler, G.J., Koutrakis, P; et al. (1989) "Exposures to Acidic Aerosols" *Environ. Health Perspect.* 79:43.

Spengler, J.D., Treitman, R.D., Tosteson, T.D., Mage, D.T., and Soczek, M.L. (1985) "Personal Exposures to Respirable Particulates and Implications for Air Pollution Epidemiology" *Environ. Sci. Tech.* 19:700–707.

Spengler, J.D. and Soczek, M.L. (1984) "Evidence for Improved Ambient Air Quality and the need for Exposure Research" *Environ. Sci. Technol.* 18:268A–280A.

Spengler, J.D., Özkaynak, H., Pellizari, E.D. and Wiener, R. (1989) "Personal Exposures to Particulate Matter: Instrumentation and Methodologies P-TEAM" Presented at the *EPA/AWMA International Symposium on Measurement of Toxic and Related Pollutants*, Raleigh, NC, May.

Spengler, J.D., Koutrakis, P., Dockery, D.W., Raizenne, M., and Speizer, F.E. (1996) "Health Effects of Acid Aerosols on North American Children: Air Pollution Exposures" *Environ. Health Perspect.* 104:492–499.

Spiegelman, J.R., Hanson, G.D. and Lazarus, A. et al. (1968) "Effect of Acute Sulphur Dioxide Exposure on Bronchial Clearance in the Donkey" *Arch. Environ. Health* 17:321.

Spix, C., Heinrich, J., Dockery D., Scwartz J., Volksch, G., Scwinkowski, K., Collen, C., and Wichamnn H.E. (1994) "Summary of the Analysis and Reanalysis Corresponding to the Publication on Air Pollution and Daily Mortality in Erfurt, E. Germany 1980–1989" *Critical Evaluation Workshop on Particulate Matter: Mortality Epidemiology Studies:* November, Raleigh, NC, USA.

Stelson A.W. and Seinfeld J.H. (1982) "Thermodynamic prediction of the water activity of NH_4NO_3 dissociation constant, density, and refractive index for the NH_4NO_3-$[NH_4]_2SO_4$-H_2O system at 25%C" *Atmos. Environ.* 16:2507–2514.

Stevens, R.K., Dzubay, T.G., Russwurm, F.R., and Rickel, D. (1978) "Sampling and analysis of atmospheric sulfates and related species" *Atmos. Environ.* 12:55.

Stevens, R.K. (1984) "Sampling and analysis of atmospheric aerosols" Presented at the *Advanced Research Workshop on Environmental Monitoring of Architectural Conservation*. NATO Science Committee. Rome, Italy.

Stidley C.A. and Samet, J.M. (1993) "A review of Ecological Studies of Lung Cancer and Indoor Radon" *Health Phys.* 65(3):234–251.

Stidley C.A. and Samet, J.M. (1994) "Assessment of Ecologic Regression in the Study of Lung Cancer and Indoor Radon" *Amer. J. Epid.* 139:312–322.

Stocks, P. (1966) "Recent epidemiological studies of lung cancer mortality, cigarette smoking, and air pollution, with discussion of a new hypothesis of causation" *Brit. J. Cancer* 20:595.

Strange, R.E. "Rapid detection of airborne microbes" In *Airborne Transmission and Airborne Infection.*, edited by J.F. Hers and K.C. Wincler, Oosthoek Publishing Co., Utrecht, The Netherlands.

Suh, H., Allen, G.A., Koutrakis, P., and Burton, R.M. (1995) "Spatial Variation in the Acidic Sulfate and Ammonia Concentrations withing Metropolitan Philadelphia" *J. Air Waste Manage. Assoc.* 45:442–452.

Suh, H., Spengler, J.D., and Koutrakis, P. (1992) "Personal Exposure to Acid Aerosols and Ammonia" *Environ. Sci. Technol.* 26:2507.

Suh, H., Koutrakis, P., and Spengler, J.D. (1993) "Validation of Personal Exposure Models for Sulfate and Aerosol Strong Acidity" *Air and Waste* 43:845.

Suh, H., Koutrakis, P., and Spengler, J.D. (1994) "The Relationship Between Airborne Acidity and Ammonia in Indoor Environments" *J. Expos. Anal. Environ. Epidemiol.* 4:2.

Sullivan, T.J. and Dickerson, M.H. (1986) "ARAC Response to the Chernobyl Reactor Accident" *Lawrence Livermore National Laboratory Report*, Livermore, CA, UCID-20834.

Sullivan, T.S., Ellis, J.S., Foster, C.S., Foster, K.T., Baskett R.L. Nasstrom, J.S, and Schalk W.W. (1994) "Modeling of Air Currents in the Gulf Region" in *The Gulf War and the Environment* Ed El-Baz and Makharita, Gordon and Breach.

Sullivan, T.S., Ellis, J.S., Foster, C.S., Foster, K.T., Baskett, R.L. Nastrom, J.S., and Schalk W. W.(1993) "Atmosperic Release Advisory Capability (ARAC): Real-Time Modeling of Airborne Hazardous Materials" *Bull. Amer. Meteor. Soc.* 74:2343–2361.

Sunyer, J., Anto, J.M., Murillo, C., and Saez, M. (1991) "Effects of urban pollution on emergency room admissions for chronic obstructive pulmonary disease" *Amer. J. Epidemiol.* 134:227–289.

Sunyer, J., Saez, M., Murillo, C., Castellsague, J., Martinez, F., and Anto, J.M. (1993) "Air pollution and emergency room admission for chronic obstructive pulmonary disease: A 5-year study" *Amer. J. Epidemiol.* 137:701–705.

Sutton, O.G. (1932) "A theory of eddy diffusion in the atmosphere" *Proc. Roy. Soc.* 135A:143.

Swift, D.L. (1989) "Direct-reading instruments for analyzing airborne particles" In *Air Sampling Instruments*, edited by S.V. Hering. American Conference of Governmental Industrial Hygienists, Inc., Cincinnati, OH.

Systems Applications Incorporated (SAI) (1987) "Effect of Power Plant NO_x emissions on Ozone Levels" EPRI EA-5333 project 1375.

Systems Applications Incorporated (SAI) (1989) "UAM" in *Urban Airshed Modelling Workshop. STAPPA/ALAPCO/EPA*, Nashville, TN. April 11–12.

Taylor, G.I. (1922) "Diffusion by Continuous Movements" *Proc. Lond Math. Soc.* 20:196–212.

Tepper J.S., Lehmann J.R., Winsett D.W., et al. (1994) "The role of surface-complexed iron in the development of acute lung inflammation and airway hyperresponsiveness" *Amer. Rev. Respir. Disease* 149:A839 (Abstract).

Thatcher, T.L. and Layton, D.W. (1995) Deposition, resuspension, and penetration of particles within residence. *Atmos. Environ.* 29:1487–1497.

Thomas, T.J. (1973) "An investigation into excess mortality and morbidity due to air pollution" Ph.D. dissertation, Purdue University, West Lafayette, Indiana.

Thurston, G.D., Ito, K., Kinney, P.L., and Lippmann, M. (1992) "A multi-year study of air pollution and respiratory hospital admissions in three New York state metropolitan areas: Results for 1988 and 1989 summers" *J. Expos. Anal. Environ. Epidemiol.* 2:429–450.

Thurston, G.D., Ito, K., and Lippmann, M. (1993) "The role of particulate mass versus acidity in the sulfate-respiratory hospital admissions association" Preprint 93–11.03. *86th Annual Meeting of the Air and Waste Management Association,* June 13–18, Denver, CO.

Thurston, G.D., Ito, K., Hayes, C.G et al. (1994) "Respiratory Hospital Admissions and Summertime Haze Air Pollution in Toronto, Ontario Cosideratio of the Role of Acid Aerosols" *Environ. Research* 65:271–290.

Thurston, G.D. and Spengler, J.D.(1985) "A Quantitative Assessment of Source Contributions to Inhaled Particulate Matter Pollution in Metropolitan Boston" *Atmos. Envir.* 19(1):9–25.

Toulomi, G., Pocock, S.J., Karsouyanni, K., and Trichopoulos D., (1994) "Short-term Effects of Air Pollution on Daily Mortality in Athens: a Time-Series Analysis" *Int. J. Epidemiol. 23:957–967.*

Turner, D.B. (1969) "Workbook of Atmospheric Dispersion Estimates" *U.S. DHEW* Washington, D.C.

Turner, W.A., Spengler, J.D., Dockery, D.W., and Colome, S.D. (1979) "Design and Performance of a Reliable Monitoring System for Respirable Particulates" *J. Air Poll. Assoc.* 29:747.

Tversky, A. and Koehler D.J., (1994) "Support Theory: A Nonextensional Representation of Subjective probability" *Psychological Review* 101:547–567.

U.S. Bureau of the Census, (1983) "1980 Census of Population" *U.S. Department of Commerce.* Washington, D.C.

Utell, M.J. (1985) "Effects of inhaled acid aerosols on lung mechanics: An analysis of human exposure studies" *Environ. Health Perspect.* 63:39–44.

Utell, M.J. and Frampton M.W. (1993) "Quantitative clinical studies with defined exposure atmospheres" In *Toxicology of the Lung.* Raven Press, New York, New York.

Utell, M.J. and Frampton M.W. (1995) "Particles and mortality: A clinical perspective" *Inhal. Toxicol.* 7:645–55.

Utell, M.J., and Mariglio J.A. (1989) "Effect of inhaled acid aerosols on respiratory function: The role of endogenous ammonia" *J. Aerosol Med.* 2:141–7.

Utell, M.J., and Morrow P.E. (1983) "Latent development of airway hyperactivity in human subjects after sulfuric acid aerosol exposure" *J. Aerosol Sci.* 14:202–5.

Utell, M.J, and Morrow, P.E. (1984) "Airway reactivity to sulfate and sulfuric acid aerosols in normal and asthmatic subjects" *J. Air Poll. Control Assoc.* 34:931–5.

Utell, M.J., Morrow, P.E., and Hyde, R.W.(1984) "Airway Reactivity to Sulfate and Sulfuric Acid Aeroso]s in Normal and Asthmatic Subjects" *J. Air Pollut. Control Assoc.* 34:931.

Utell, M.J., Morrow, P.E., Speers, D.M., et al. (1983) "Airway responses to sulfate and sulfuric acid aerosols in asthmatics" *Amer. Rev. Respir. Disease* 128:444–50.

Utell, M.J., and Samet, J.M., (1993) "Particulate air pollution and health. New evidence on an old problem" *Amer. Rev. Resp. Disease* 147:1334–1335.

Verhoff, A.P., Hoek, G., Scwartz, J. and van Wijuen J.H. (1996) "Air Pollution and Daily Mortality in Amsterdam, the Netherlands" *Epidemiology* 7:in press.

Wacholder, S. (1995) "When Measurement Errors Correlate with Truth: Surprising Effects of Nondifferential Misclassification" *Epidemiology* 6:157–161.

Wallace, L. (1987) "The Total Exposure Assessment Methodology (TEAM) Study" EPA/600/6-87/002a.

Wallace, L., Pellizzari, E., Hartwell, T.D., Perritt, R., and Ziengenfus, R. (1987) "Exposures to benzene and other volatile organic compounds from active and passive smoking" *Arch. Environ. Health* 42(5):272–279.

Wallace, L., Nelson, W., Ziegenfus, R., Pellizzari, E., Michael, L., Whitmore, R., Zelon, H., Hartwell, T., Perritt, R., and Westerdahl, D. (1991) "The Los Angeles TEAM study: Personal exposures, indoor-outdoor air concentrations, and breath concentrations of 25 volative organic compounds" *J. Expos. Anal. Environ. Epidemiol.* 1(2):157–192.

Wallace, L., (1996) "Indoor Particles: A Review" *J. Air Waste Manage. Assoc.* 46:98–126.

Waller R.E. and Swan, A.V. (1992) "Invited commentary: Particulate air pollution and daily mortality" *Amer. J. Epidemiol.* 135:20–22.

Wang, A. (1981) "Chemical characteristics of airborne particles in the Beijing area" *Acta Scientiae Circumstantiae* (in Chinese) 1:220.

Wang H.C. and John W. (1988) "Characteristics of the Berner impactor for sampling inorganic ions" *Aerosol Sci. & Technol.* 8(2):157–172.

Ware, J.H., Thibodeau, L.A., Speizer, F.E., Colome, S., and Ferris, Jr., B.G. (1981) "Assessment of the health effects of atmospheric sulfur oxides and particulate matter: Evidence from observational studies" *Environ. Health Perspect.* 41:255–276.

Warren, D.L. and Last, J.A. (1987) "Synergistic Interaction of Ozone and Respirable Aerosols on Rat Lungs. III. Ozone and Sulfuric Acid" *Toxicol. Appl. Pharmacol.* 88:203.

Wheeler T.A., Horn, S.C., Cramond, W.R., and Unwin S.D. (1989) "Analyis of Core Damage Frequency from Intenal Events: Expert Judgement Elicitation" *NUREG/CR4550; SANDIA 2084 v2* US Nuclear Regulatory Commission, Washington, D.C.

Whitby, K.T., and Cantrell, B.K. (1975) "Atmospheric Aerosols: Characteristics and Measurements" International Conference on *Environmental Sensing and Assessment* IEEE, Las Vegas, NV.

Whitby, K.T. (1976) "Electrical measurement of aerosols" In *Fine Particles*, edited by B.Y.H. Liu, Academic Press, New York.

Whitby, K.T. and Svendrup, G.M. (1980) "California Aerosols: Their Physical and Chemical Characteristics" *Adv. Environ. Sci. Tech.* 10:477.

Whitby, K.T., Cantrell, B.K., and Kittelson, D.B. (1978) "Nuclei formation rates in a coal-fired power plant plume" *Atmos. Environ.* 12:313–322.

Whittemore, A.S., and Korn, E.L. (1980) "Asthma and air pollution in the Los Angeles Area" *Amer. J. Public Health* 70:687–696.

WHO (1960) World Health Organization Technical Report Ser. 192.

WHO (1962) "Epidemiology of Air Pollution" Geneva: World Health Organization Public Health Paper No. 15.

WMO (1992) "Report of the Second WMO Meeting of Experts to Assess the Response to, and Atmospheric Effects of, the Kuwait Oil Fires" World Meteorological Organization, Geneva, Switzerland, 25–29 May.

Wichmann, H.E., Mueller, W. Allhoff, P. et al. (1989) "Health effects during a smog episode in West Germany in 1985" *Environ. Health Perspect.* 79:89–99.

Willeke, K. and Liu, B.Y.H. (1976) "Single particle optical counters: principle and applications" In *Fine Particles*, edited by B.Y.H. Liu, Academic Press, New York.

Wilkins E.T. (1953) "Air Pollution Aspects of the London Fog of December 1952" *Quarterly J. Roy. Meteor. Soc.* 80:267–271.

Wilson R., Colome, S.D., Spengler, J.D., and Wilson D.G. (1980) "Health Effects of Fossil Fuel Burning: Assessment and Mitigation" *Ballinger,* Cambridge, MA.

Wyzga, R.E. 1978. "The effect of air pollution on mortality—A consideration of distributed lag models" *J. Amer. Stat. Assoc.* 73:463–72.

Xue, J., Özkaynak, H., Ware, J.H., Spengler, J.D., Billick, I.H. and Silvers, A. (1993) "Alternative estimates of exposure to nitrogen dioxide and their implications to epidemiologic study design" *Presented at Indoor Air '93* Helsinki, Finland, July.

Xu, X., Dockery, D., and Wang, L. (1991) "Effects of Air Pollution on Adult Pulmonary Function" *Arch. Environ. Health* 46:198–206.

Xu, X., Gao, J., Dockery, D., and Chen, Y. (1994) "Air Pollution and Daily Mortality in Residential Areas of Beijing, China" *Arch. Environ. Health* 49:216–222.

Xu, X., Dockery, D., Christiani, D., Li, B., and Huang, H. (1995a) "Association of Air Pollution with Hospital Outpatient Visits in Beijing" *Arch. Environ. Health* In press.

Xu, X.P., Dockery, D.W., Ware, J.H., Speizer, F.E., and Ferris, B.G., Jr. (1992) "Effects of Cigarette Smoking on Rate of Loss of Pulmonary Function in Adults: A Longitudinal Assessment" *Amer. Rev. Resp. Disease* 146:1345–1348.

Yocom, J.E., Clink, W.L. and Cote, W.A. (1971) "Indoor/Outdoor Air Quality Relationships" *J. Air Poll. Control Assoc.* 21:251.

Yocom, J.E., (1982) "Indoor-Outdoor Air Quality Relationships: A Critical Review" *J. Air Poll. Control Assoc.* 32:500.

Addendum

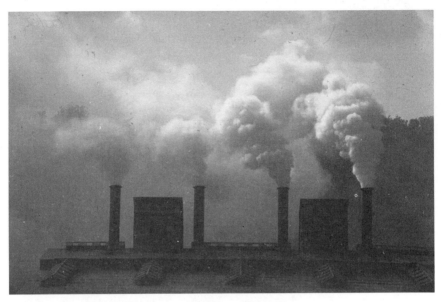

Foundry along Ohio River near Stubenville, OH.
Photo: J. Spengler or D. Dockery

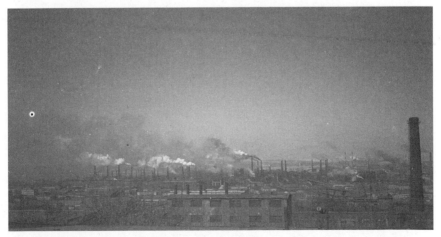

The steel town of Magnitogorsk, Ural mountains, Russia from the east.
Photo: R. Wilson

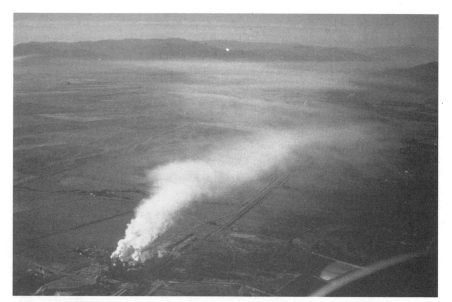

Copper smelter in American Southwest showing long distance transport in stable air. Photo: W. Zoller

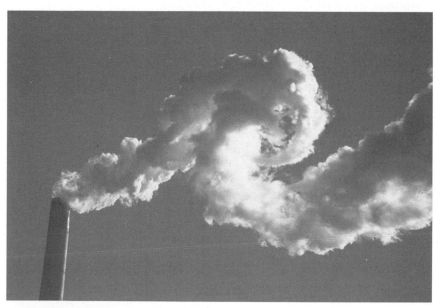

Plume from a Boston Edison electricity generating plant showing "looping in unstable air. Photo: J. Spengler

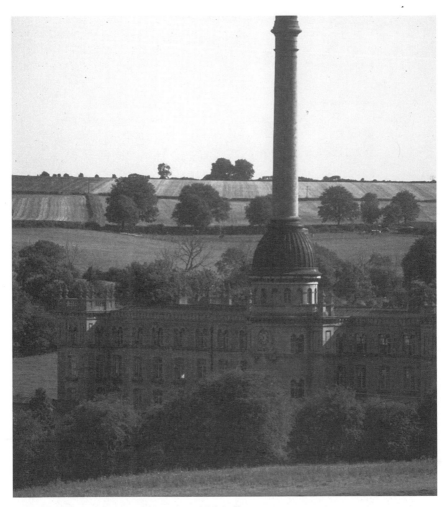

Old factory in the English Cotswold hills. Photo D. Burg

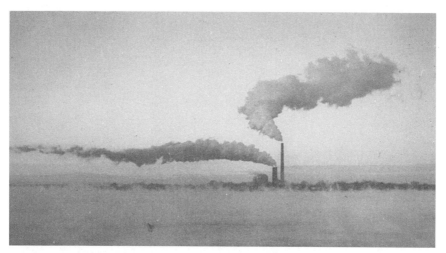

Condensation plumes from 75 meter and 100 meter stacks in Salem, MA, showing effect of windshear and ground fog. Photo: R Turcotte

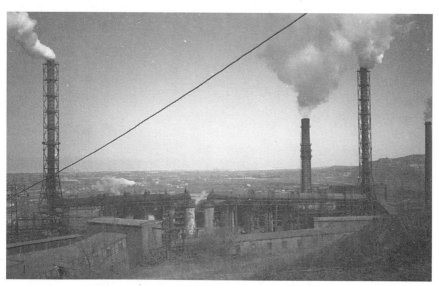

Ore reduction plant at Magnitogorsk, Russia. Photo: R Wilson

Index